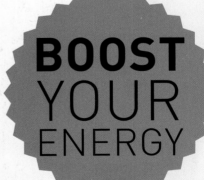

BUILD MUSCLE

BURN FAT

BOOST YOUR ENERGY

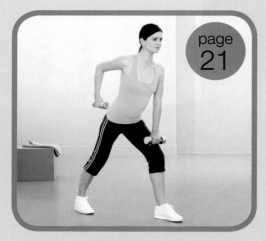

page 21

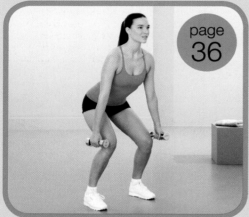

page 36

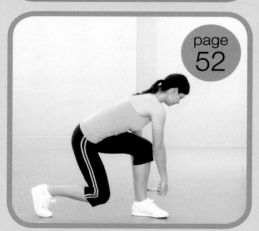

page 52

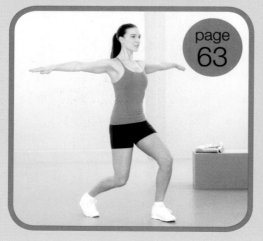

page 63

Contents

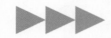

Getting started

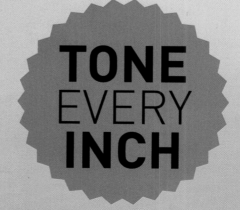

TONE
EVERY
INCH

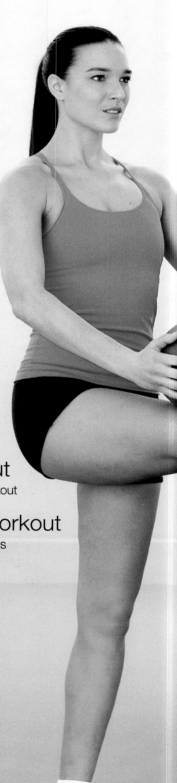

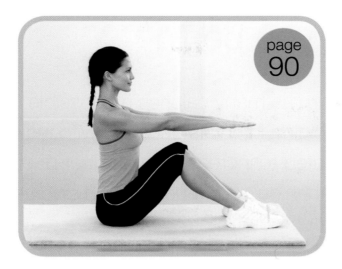

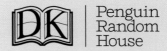

page
90

Focus on...

DK | Penguin Random House

Consultant Joan Pagano
Project Editor Elizabeth Yeates
Designer Alison Shackleton
Senior Jacket Creative Mark Penfound
Pre-Production Producer Rebecca Fallowfield
Senior Producer Charlotte Oliver
Special Sales Creative Project Manager
Alison Donovan

Health warning: All participants in fitness activities must assume the responsibility for their own actions and safety. If you have any health problems or medical conditions, consult your doctor before undertaking any of the activities set out in this book. The information contained in this book cannot replace sound judgement and good decision making, which can help reduce risk of injury.

First published in Great Britain in 2015
by Dorling Kindersley Limited
80 Strand, London WC2R 0RL

Material previously published in:
Strength Training for Women (2013), Get Fit for Summer Flat Tum (2014), Get Fit for Summer Skinny Jeans (2014), Get Fit for Summer Stretching (2014), Get Fit for Summer Toned Bum (2014)

A CIP catalogue record for this book is available from the British Library.
ISBN 978-0-2412-1658-3

Printed and bound in Italy by L.E.G.O S.p.A.

All images © Dorling Kindersley Limited
For further information see: www.dkimages.com

A WORLD OF IDEAS
SEE ALL THERE IS TO KNOW

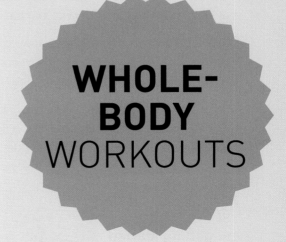

WHOLE-BODY WORKOUTS

The key to getting fit fast is to burn as many calories as possible while sculpting lean muscles. By combining intervals of cardio with resistance exercises, your heart rate is elevated to increase the number of calories you burn, simultaneously strengthening your muscles with diverse patterns of stress to speed up your metabolism.

Body composition, one of the health-related aspects of physical fitness, is the 'quality' of your weight as opposed to the 'quantity' of your weight measured by the scales. You can gauge your body-fat status roughly by the fit of a favourite pair of jeans. One pound (0.5 kg) of fat takes up more space than 1 pound (0.5 kg) of muscle, so as you lose fat, you literally shrink.

▶▶▶ **safety** notes

● When lifting weights, concentrate on proper form and alignment, stabilizing the core body before you lift. Coordinate the movement with your breath: inhale first, then exhale as you lift the weight.

● If you find an exercise too difficult, just do the lower-body movement at first.

● **A word of caution for the knees:** Form is especially important when performing squats and lunges, which can be tough on weak knees. When doing a squat, keep your weight back on your heels so that when you bend your legs, your knees stay behind your toes.

● Do not allow your hips to drop below your knees. There is a forward lean to the torso but your spine should remain straight, with a natural curve in the low back.

● When performing a lunge, again make sure that your front knee stays behind your toes (keep a right angle at the knee). Do not allow momentum to push your knee forward, as this creates instability in the knee joint which can cause stress.

A combination of cardio activity and strength training is the key for reducing fat (of course combined with a healthy diet!). Cardio activity burns calories and shrinks fat cells from the entire body. Strength-training revs up the metabolism by building lean body mass (muscle), so you continue to burn calories throughout the day. Resistance training (also referred to as weight training or weight lifting) is the technique of applying resistance to the muscles in order to stimulate development. The resistance can be your own body weight as well as free weights used in the workouts. Lifting weights will sculpt the contours of your body. As you work your muscles, they become more defined. You will have a flatter tummy, a shapelier bum and firmer thighs.

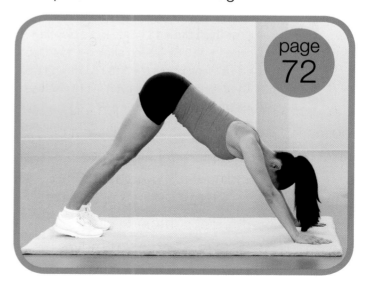

page
72

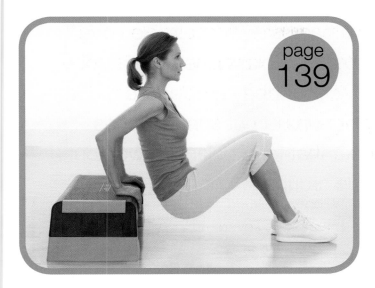

page
139

Here, the workouts combine cardio and strength training to tone you all over. Each programme begins with a three-minute warm up sequence that gradually builds in intensity. The main body of the workout is comprised of 10 minutes of resistance training exercises for the major muscle groups alternating with cardio intervals. The sequence ends with a two-minute cool down, providing full body stretches. Each routine takes 15 minutes and can all be carried out at home. If you want even faster results, you can combine the workouts for a longer workout.

The programmes are designed with increasing difficulty to help you progress as you become more fit. If you are just beginning, gently ease yourself into the habit of exercising with Step-touch. When this routine feels too easy, move onto Beach ball, which requires more coordination and balance while adding variety to your workout with a ball. Hop, jig, and jump is yet more vigorous, while Lunge around the clock challenges you with more complex moves to advance your skills and fitness level.

After the workouts is the focused exercises. These offer you the option of adding additional exercises to target typical female trouble spots – the tum, bum and thighs, arms and back. After you finish your 15-minute full-body workout, pick 8-10 of the focused exercises from one of these categories. This will focus your efforts on a target zone where you wish to see extra toning. Perform one to two sets of each exercise for 10 repetitions. When you feel ready, progress by increasing the number of reps to 12–15, or using heavier weights. Always do the stretches at the end of the section.

Step-by-step photos show you how to do the exercises. The inset photos give you the starting position for the exercises, when necessary. The large photographs give you the steps required to complete it.

Have two sets of weights ready; if you are just starting to lift weights, or are returning after a long absence, use lighter weights, 3–5lb (1–2kg). If you are already experienced with weights or are ready to progress from the lighter weight, use heavier weights, 8–10lb (4–5kg).

Do your workout 3 to 4 times a week, with a day of rest in between. The rest is as important for muscle development as the stress. It allows the muscle time to recover and rebuild. This is when the fitness gains occur, not as you are doing the exercise.

Joan Pagano

If you know which muscle is working in a particular exercise, you can enhance your effort by mentally focusing on it. This will help you key into the muscular movement and improve your body awareness. The anatomical illustrations below will help you target specific areas that you want to work on – but remember that for a balanced workout, you need to work on all the major muscle groups.

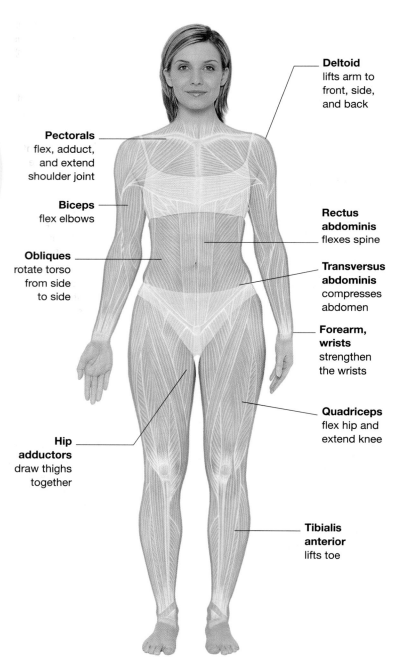

Lifting weights will make you bulk up

This is true only if you have high levels of testosterone and use very heavy weights. Most women lack the necessary hormones and strength to build muscle mass. Female body builders are genetically predisposed to build big muscles; they also follow rigorous exercise and diet regimens to maximize their muscle size. The average woman who lifts weights actually shrinks in body size by losing fat and shaping the muscles.

You shouldn't lift weights if you are an older adult, overweight, or out of shape

Not so! Weight training can help you rejuvenate, boost metabolism, lose weight, and shape up. Begin with 4–6 simple exercises that you find manageable and gradually progress by increasing the level of difficulty and adding exercises.

Deltoid
lifts arm to front, side, and back

Pectorals
flex, adduct, and extend shoulder joint

Biceps
flex elbows

Rectus abdominis
flexes spine

Obliques
rotate torso from side to side

Transversus abdominis
compresses abdomen

Forearm, wrists
strengthen the wrists

Quadriceps
flex hip and extend knee

Hip adductors
draw thighs together

Tibialis anterior
lifts toe

A thin person does not need to build lean body mass by lifting weights
Appearances are deceiving when it comes to body composition, and being thin is no guarantee that you are lean. Without weight training, you steadily lose muscle and gain fat as you age.

Certain weight-training exercises can help you spot reduce
You can spot strengthen and shape a body area, but fat belongs to the whole body and needs to be reduced all over, through expending more calories than you consume. High-repetition training will keep the hips trim, while using heavier weights to strengthen the upper body can make your hips look more in balance.

Aerobic activities, not weight training, are the most efficient type of exercise to lose weight
Losing weight requires a balanced exercise programme of aerobic exercise to burn calories and weight training to speed up the metabolism.

A 15-minute workout won't make a difference to your health and weight
The key is consistency. Brief doses of exercise done consistently over time are effective at reducing the risk of developing chronic diseases such as diabetes and hypertension. They also have a positive effect on appearance, reducing fat, and increasing muscle tone and flexibility.

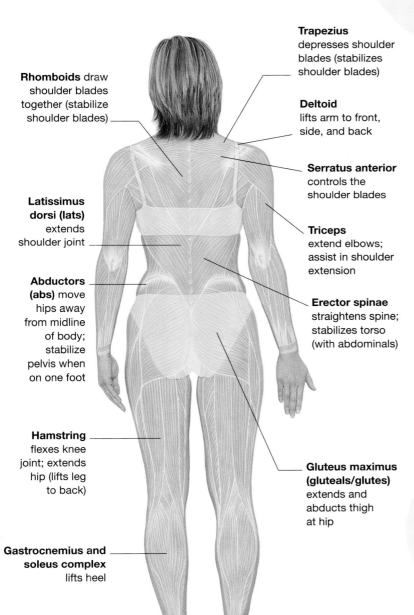

Rhomboids draw shoulder blades together (stabilize shoulder blades)

Latissimus dorsi (lats) extends shoulder joint

Abductors (abs) move hips away from midline of body; stabilize pelvis when on one foot

Hamstring flexes knee joint; extends hip (lifts leg to back)

Gastrocnemius and soleus complex lifts heel

Trapezius depresses shoulder blades (stabilizes shoulder blades)

Deltoid lifts arm to front, side, and back

Serratus anterior controls the shoulder blades

Triceps extend elbows; assist in shoulder extension

Erector spinae straightens spine; stabilizes torso (with abdominals)

Gluteus maximus (gluteals/glutes) extends and abducts thigh at hip

▶▶▶ **your body** composition

A well-toned figure is something that we all aspire to, but body composition and shape are about more than just appearance: they are also closely related to fitness and health. Three simple measures are used to assess whether your body fat distribution is in a healthy range – apple and pear concept, waist-to-hip ratio, and body mass index (BMI).

Track your progress

Studies show that a large waist circumference signals a greater risk of heart disease, high blood pressure, and diabetes, than ample hips and thighs. This relationship between body shape and disease is sometimes summed up by the concept of "apples and pears": a person who tends to gain weight around the middle is described as apple-shaped, while one whose fat tends to settle around the hips and thighs is said to be pear-shaped. People with apple-shaped figures are at increased risk of the diseases associated with abdominal obesity. Although your body type is inherited, you can minimize the associated health risks by controlling your weight and keeping fit.

Another simple way to determine body-fat distribution is the waist-to-hip ratio. In women aged 20–39, a ratio of more than .79 is considered high; for women aged 40–59, the figure is .82; and for those aged 60–69, it is .84.

Body Mass Index (BMI), based on a ratio of weight to height, is used to assess the increased risk of weight-related health conditions. It may be inaccurate in some cases—for example, for someone with a lot of muscle mass, as muscle weighs more than fat—but the chart opposite is a simple way to check whether your weight is within healthy limits. Look down the column on the left-hand side of the table to find your weight (or the nearest to it); then look across that row until you see the column for your height. The number that appears where the two meet is your BMI score. If the result indicates that your weight poses a health risk, seek advice from your doctor.

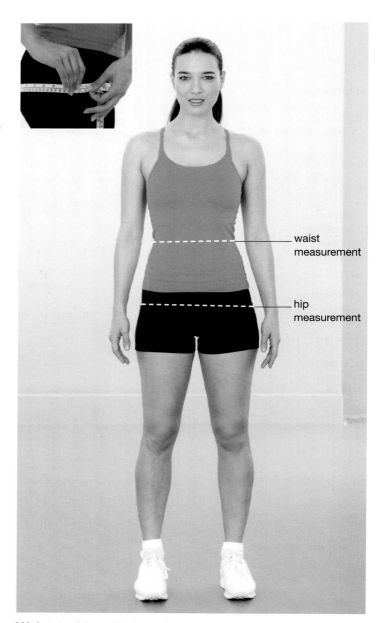

waist
measurement

hip
measurement

Waist-to-hip ratio is a simple way to determine whether your body-fat distribution poses a health risk to you. Divide your waist measurement by your hip measurement to calculate the ratio.

Check your Body Mass Index (BMI)

Weight	Height 1.46m (4ft 9in)	1.52m (4ft 11in)	1.58m (5ft 2in)	1.62m (5ft 4in)	1.68m (5ft 6in)	1.74m (5ft 8in)	1.78m (5ft 10in)	1.82m (5ft 11in)	1.88m (6ft 2in)	1.94m (6ft 4in)
50kg (110lb)	23	22	20	19	18	17	16	15	14	13
52kg (115lb)	24	23	21	20	18	17	16	16	15	14
54kg (120lb)	25	24	22	21	19	18	17	16	15	15
57kg (125lb)	26	24	23	22	20	19	18	17	16	15
59kg (130lb)	27	25	24	22	21	20	19	18	17	16
61kg (135lb)	28	26	25	23	22	21	19	18	17	16
63kg (140lb)	29	27	26	24	23	21	20	19	18	17
66kg (145lb)	30	28	27	25	23	22	21	20	19	18
68kg (150lb)	31	29	28	26	24	23	22	20	19	18
70kg (155lb)	32	30	28	27	25	24	22	21	20	19
73kg (160lb)	34	31	29	28	26	24	23	22	21	20
75kg (165lb)	35	32	30	28	27	25	24	22	21	20
77kg (170lb)	36	33	31	29	28	26	24	23	22	21
79kg (175lb)	37	34	32	30	28	27	25	24	23	21
82kg (180lb)	38	35	33	31	29	27	26	24	23	22
84kg (185lb)	39	36	34	32	30	28	27	25	24	23
86kg (190lb)	40	37	35	33	31	29	27	26	24	23
88kg (195lb)	41	38	36	34	32	30	28	27	25	24
91kg (200lb)	42	39	37	34	32	30	29	27	26	24
93kg (205lb)	43	40	38	35	33	31	29	28	26	25
95kg (210lb)	44	41	39	36	34	32	30	29	27	26
98kg (215lb)	45	42	39	37	35	33	31	29	28	26
100kg (220lb)	46	43	40	38	36	34	32	30	28	27
102kg (225lb)	47	44	41	39	36	34	32	31	29	27
104kg (230lb)	48	45	42	40	37	35	33	31	30	28
107kg (235lb)	49	46	43	40	38	36	34	32	30	29
109kg (240lb)	50	47	44	41	39	37	35	33	31	29
111kg (245lb)	51	48	45	42	40	37	35	33	32	30

What does your score mean?

Below 18.5 — You are underweight, which may signal malnutrition

18.6–24.9 — You are within a healthy weight range for your height

25–29.9 — You are overweight, with an increased risk of health problems

30 and above — You are obese, with a significantly increased risk of health problems

Before you start your training programme, you must check that it is safe for you to begin. Take the PAR-Q questionnaire on the opposite page, and if you are in any doubt about the state of your health, please see your doctor before becoming more physically active. The four tests below will help you to assess your fitness.

Track your progress

One way to measure muscular fitness is to count how many repetitions you can perform, or how many seconds you can hold a contraction. To see how you measure up, do the four exercises shown, which will assess your muscular endurance in the upper, middle, lower, and core body. Record your results, noting the date, and after three months of training, repeat the tests. When you reassess yourself, perform the same version of the exercise.

If you are just beginning to exercise, or coming back to it after a long break, you may prefer to perform your first assessment after two or three months of exercising on a regular basis. Before attempting the exercises, warm up first by moving your arms and legs briskly for 5 minutes.

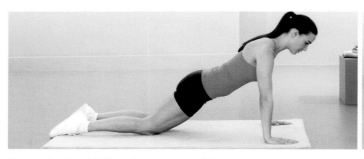

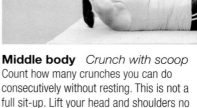

Upper body *Half push-up*
Inhale as you bend your elbows, lowering your chest to the floor. Exhale as you push up to the start position. Count how many half push-ups you can do consecutively without resting.

Your score	
Excellent	20 reps or more
Good	15–19 reps
Fair	10–14 reps
Poor	10 reps or fewer

Middle body *Crunch with scoop*
Count how many crunches you can do consecutively without resting. This is not a full sit-up. Lift your head and shoulders no higher than 30 degrees off the mat.

Your score	
Excellent	50 reps or more
Good	35–49 reps
Fair	20–34 reps
Poor	20 reps or fewer

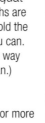

Lower body *Wall squat*
Slide down until your thighs are parallel to the floor and hold the position for as long as you can. (If you cannot slide all the way down, go as far as you can.)

Your score	
Excellent	90 seconds or more
Good	60 seconds
Fair	30 seconds
Poor	less than 30 seconds

Core body *Forearm plank*
From a kneeling position, bend your elbows under your shoulders, hands in loose fists. Straighten one leg behind you, then the other. Tighten your abdominals to keep your torso lifted in a straight line from shoulders to heels. Hold the position, breathing naturally.

Your score	
Excellent	90 seconds or more
Good	60 seconds
Fair	30 seconds
Poor	less than 30 seconds

 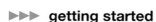

PAR-Q & YOU (a questionnaire for people aged 15–69)

Regular physical activity is fun and healthy, and increasingly more people are starting to become more active every day. Being more active is very safe for most people. However, some people should check with their doctor before they start becoming much more physically active.

If you are planning to become much more physically active than you are now, start by answering the seven questions in the box below. If you are between the ages of 15 and 69, the PAR-Q will tell you if you should check with your doctor before you start. If you are over 69 years of age, and you are not used to being very active, check with your doctor.

Common sense is your best guide when you answer these questions. Please read the questions carefully and answer each one honestly: check YES or NO.

YES NO

☐ ☐ **1** Has your doctor ever said that you have a heart condition <u>and</u> that you should only do physical activity recommended by a doctor?

☐ ☐ **2** Do you feel pain in your chest when you do physical activity?

☐ ☐ **3** In the past month, have you had chest pain when you were not doing physical activity?

☐ ☐ **4** Do you lose your balance because of dizziness or do you ever lose consciousness?

YES NO

☐ ☐ **5** Do you have a bone or joint problem (for example, back, knee, or hip) that could be made worse by a change in your physical activity?

☐ ☐ **6** Is your doctor currently prescribing drugs (for example, water pills) for your blood pressure or heart condition?

☐ ☐ **7** Do you know of <u>any other reason</u> why you should not do physical activity?

If you answered YES to one or more questions

Talk with your doctor by phone or in person BEFORE you start becoming much more physically active or BEFORE you have a fitness appraisal.
Tell your doctor about the PAR-Q and which questions you answered YES to.
• You may be able to do any activity you want – as long as you start slowly and build up gradually. Or, you may need to restrict your activities to those which are safe for you. Talk with your doctor about the kinds of activities you wish to participate in and follow his/her advice.
• Find out which community programmes are safe and helpful for you.

If you answered NO to all questions

If you answered NO honestly to all PAR-Q questions, you can be reasonably sure that you can:
• start becoming much more physically active – begin slowly and build up gradually. This is the safest and easiest way to go.
• take part in a fitness appraisal – this is an excellent way to determine your basic fitness so that you can plan the best way for you to live actively. It is also highly recommended that you have your blood pressure evaluated. If your reading is over 144/94, talk with your doctor before you start becoming much more physically active.

DELAY BECOMING MUCH MORE ACTIVE:
• if you are not feeling well because of a temporary illness such as a cold or a fever – wait until you feel better; or

• if you are or may be pregnant – talk to your doctor before you start becoming more active.

PLEASE NOTE:
If your health changes so that you then answer YES to any of the above questions, tell your fitness or health professional. Ask whether you should change your physical activity plan.

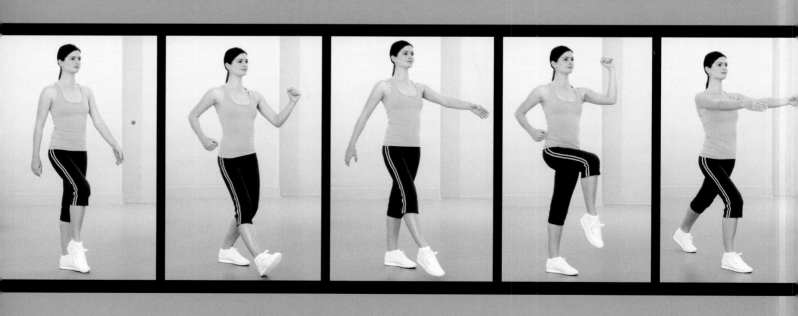

get moving

step-touch
workout

Gently ease yourself into the habit of
exercising with this lighter workout.
Grab some light free weights and begin!

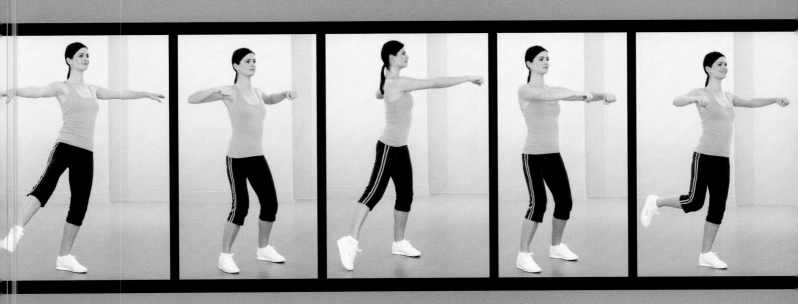

1 **March** Stand with your feet parallel, hip width apart, knees soft, arms by your sides. Begin marching, bending one knee to bring the foot just off the floor and swinging the opposite arm forwards and other arm back. Step down on the ball of your foot, rolling through to the heel. Continue marching, using opposite arm/leg action. Repeat for a total of 8 reps (1 rep = both sides).

2 **Heel dig** Continuing to march, change the foot pattern to a heel dig to the front. Extend your leg to the front, knee straight, heel to the floor, toe to the ceiling. Continue to pump the arms in opposition as you march, with elbows bent close to your sides, raising the front fist to shoulder height. Remember to keep your abdominals pulled tight. Repeat for a total of 8 reps (1 rep = both sides).

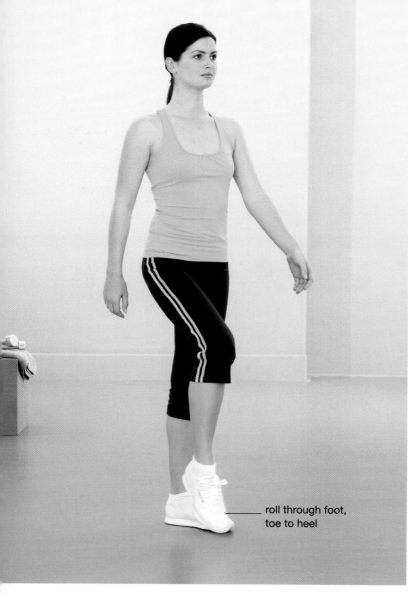

roll through foot, toe to heel

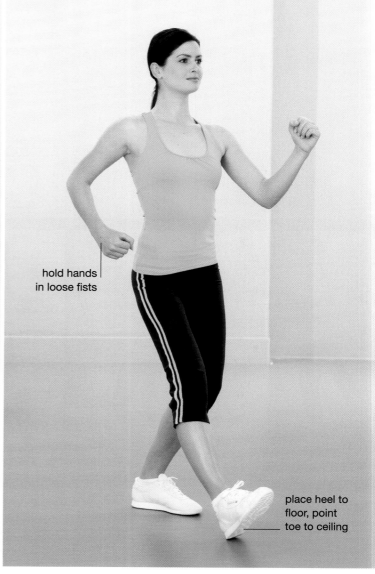

hold hands in loose fists

place heel to floor, point toe to ceiling

3 **Toe reach** Change the foot pattern to a toe reach to the front and continue marching, alternating feet and arms. As you extend your leg, point the foot, lengthening from toe to hip. Keep your arms straight as you swing them, raising the front hand to shoulder height. As you work, focus on your alignment. Stack your shoulders over your hips, over your ankles. Look straight ahead. Repeat the Toe Reach for a total of 8 reps (1 rep = both sides).

4 **Knee raise** Step up the intensity by bending the front knee to hip height. If you are able to lift the knee higher than your hip, be sure to use your core muscles to maintain proper alignment. Continue to pump the arms in opposition, raising the front elbow to shoulder level. Repeat the Knee raise for a total of 8 reps (1 rep = both sides).

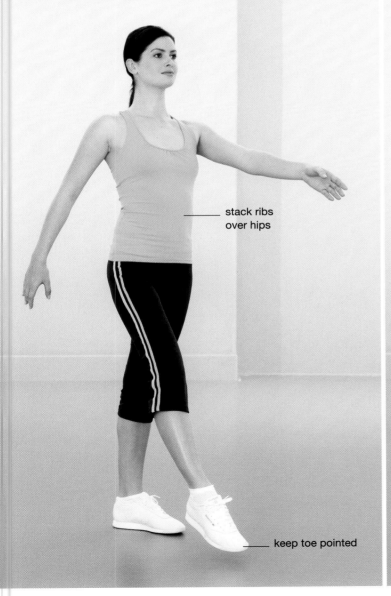

stack ribs over hips

keep toe pointed

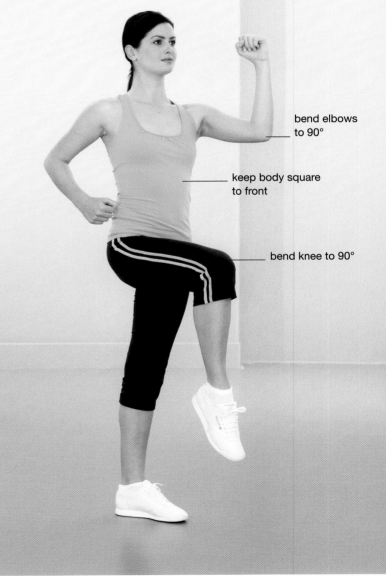

bend elbows to 90°

keep body square to front

bend knee to 90°

5 **Reverse lunge** Maintaining the same rhythm, bend one leg and extend the the other leg behind, heel raised. Raise both arms to the front at shoulder height. Push off with the ball of your back foot to return to centre, arms returning to your sides, then switch sides and repeat. Repeat the Reverse Lunge for a total of 8 reps (1 rep = both sides).

6 **Lateral lift** Maintaining the same rhythm, bend both knees, arms by your sides. Then straighten both legs, lift one leg to the side and raise both arms to shoulder level. Return the raised leg to centre, knees bent. Repeat, alternating sides, for 8 reps (1 rep = both sides). Now **reverse the warm up**, starting with Step 5, and working back through Steps 4, 3, and 2, and finishing with Step 1, marching in place.

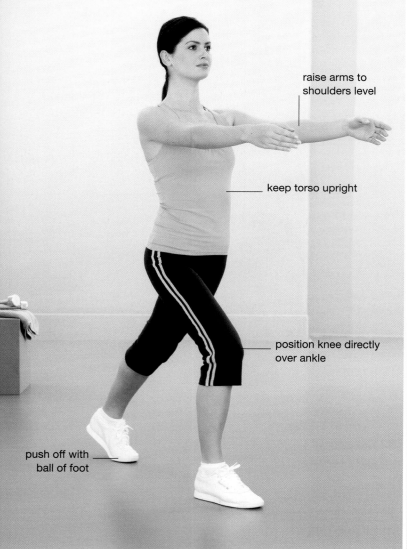

raise arms to shoulders level

keep torso upright

position knee directly over ankle

push off with ball of foot

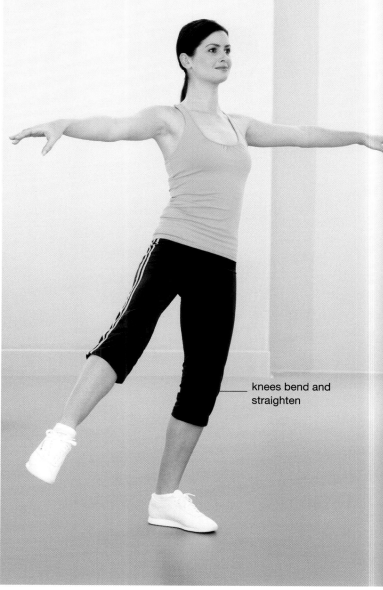

knees bend and straighten

7a **Plié with lateral raise** Pick up two small free weights and stand with your feet in a wide stance. Shift your weight to your heels and turn your legs out from the hips as a unit until your feet are at 45° angles. Hold the free weights with palms facing in, arms straight by your sides. Remember to pull your abdominals tight and draw your shoulder blades down and together.

7b Inhale as you bend your knees in line with your feet, lifting your arms out to the sides to shoulder height, thumbs up to the ceiling. Angle your arms slightly forward of your body, directly above your thighs. Keep your elbows slightly rounded and your wrists straight. Exhale and press through your heels as you straighten your legs and lower your arms to return to the start position. As you move, imagine you are sliding up and down a wall. Repeat for a total of 12 reps.

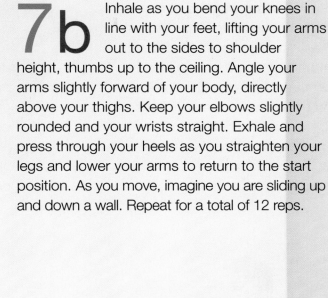

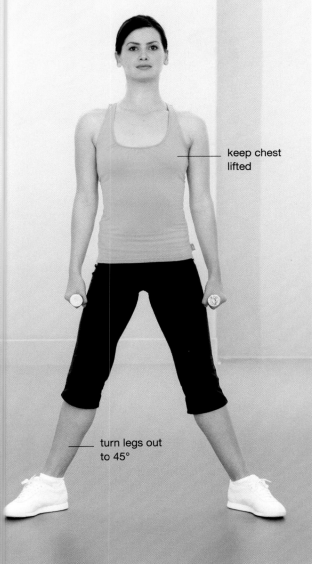

keep chest lifted

turn legs out to 45°

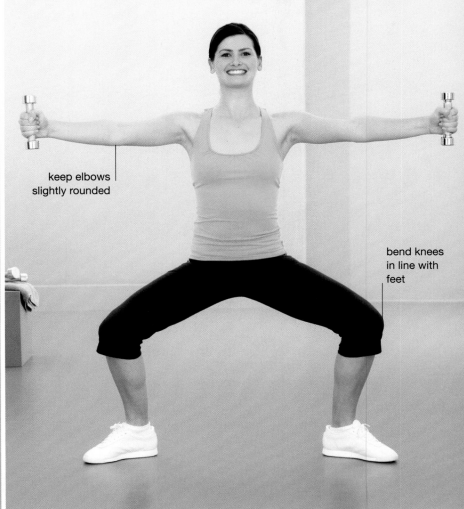

keep elbows slightly rounded

bend knees in line with feet

8 a **Step & punch** Put down the weights for the first cardio interval. Stand with your feet parallel, shoulder width apart, knees bent in a demi plié. Bend your arms and hold them at shoulder height, hands in loose fists. Check your alignment: keep your shoulder blades down, abdominals tight, chest lifted, and torso square to the front.

8 b Breathe in, then exhale as you straighten your knees and extend one arm diagonally across your body (like a punch), at the same time lifting the heel of the same leg. Keep your other arm bent at shoulder height. Inhale as you return to the start position and repeat, alternating sides, for 12 reps (1 rep = both sides).

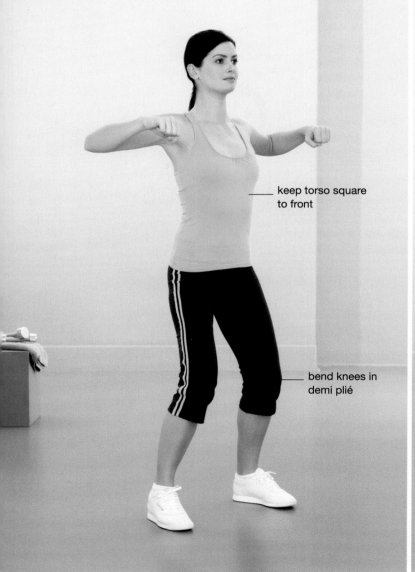

keep torso square to front

bend knees in demi plié

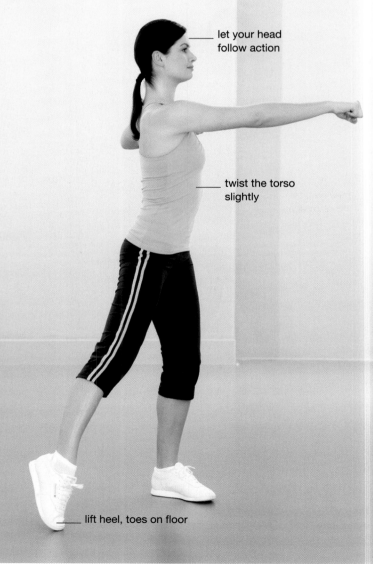

let your head follow action

twist the torso slightly

lift heel, toes on floor

9a **Curl & squeeze** Stand with your feet parallel, shoulder width apart, knees soft. Raise your arms to the front at shoulder level, shoulder width apart, hands in loose fists, palms down. Keep your knees soft. Use your core muscles to maintain neutral spine alignment, and lower your shoulder blades as you prepare to work the muscles of the mid-back.

9b Breathing naturally throughout, shift your weight onto one leg and simultaneously bend the other leg back, heel toward your buttocks, in a hamstring curl. Keep your arms parallel to the floor, elbows bent at 90°, as you squeeze your shoulder blades together. Inhale as you return to the starting position. Repeat, alternating legs, for a total of 8 reps (1 rep = both sides).

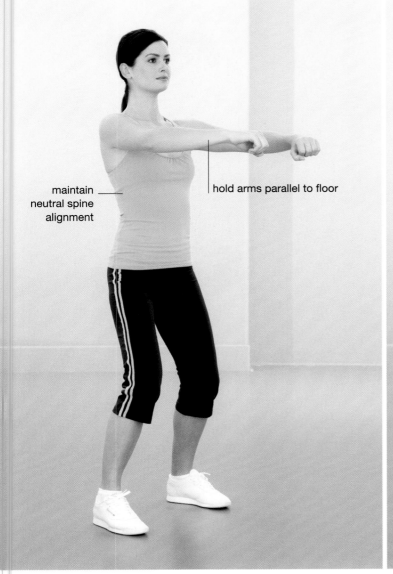

maintain neutral spine alignment

hold arms parallel to floor

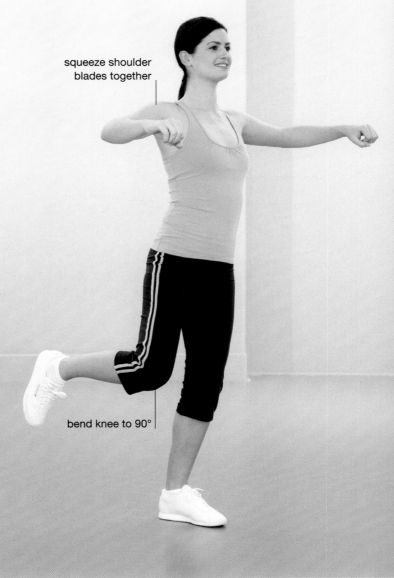

squeeze shoulder blades together

bend knee to 90°

10a

Twisting knee lift Stand with your feet parallel, hip width apart, knees soft. Raise your arms out to the sides at shoulder height and bend your elbows to 90°; with palms facing forwards, make your hands into loose fists. Remember to keep your shoulder blades down and abdominals pulled tight as you get ready to twist.

10b

Keeping your back straight, bend your knee to hip height. Exhale and rotate your torso through the centre to bring your elbow towards your raised knee. Inhale as you return to the centre and repeat, alternating sides, for 8 reps (1 rep = both sides).

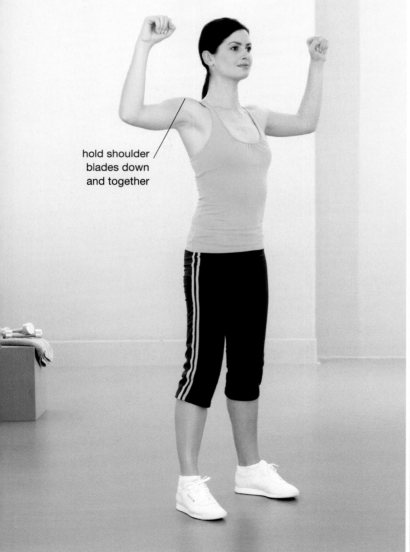

hold shoulder blades down and together

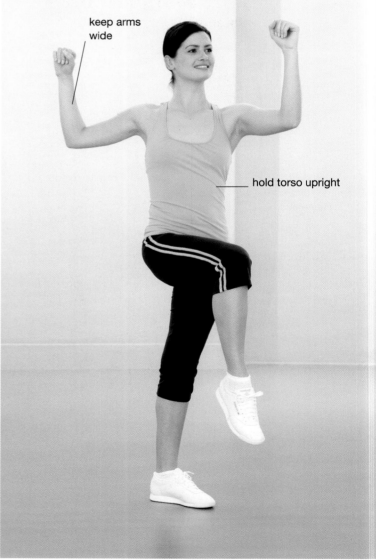

keep arms wide

hold torso upright

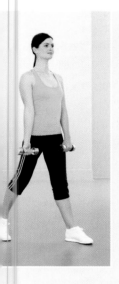

11 **Lunge & curl** Pick up two large free weights. Stand in a staggered lunge position, one foot forwards. Hold the weight in your opposite hand, palm forwards. Inhale as you bend your knees into a lunge and bend one elbow to raise the weight to shoulder height. Exhale to return to centre. Do 12 reps on each side (1 rep = both sides). **Do your next cardio interval, Steps 8–10.**

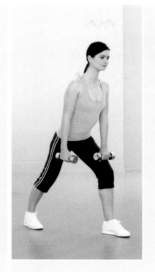

12 **One-arm row** Pick up two large free weights and step into a staggered lunge, bending from the hip to 45°. Inhale as you bend the opposite elbow behind you to 90°, lifting the weight to waist height. Do 12 reps on both sides. **Now do your next cardio interval, Steps 8–10.**

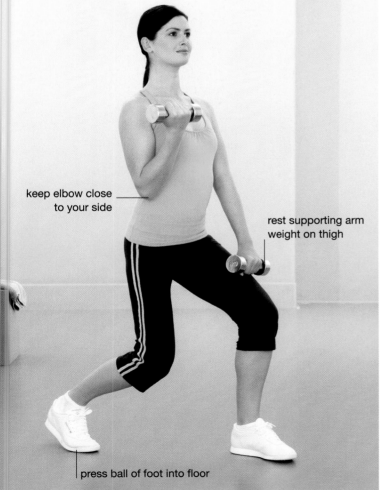

keep elbow close to your side

rest supporting arm weight on thigh

press ball of foot into floor

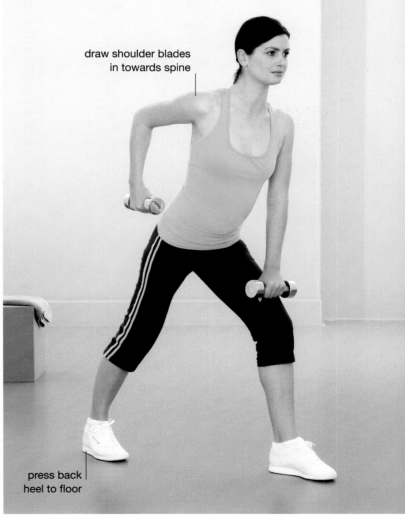

draw shoulder blades in towards spine

press back heel to floor

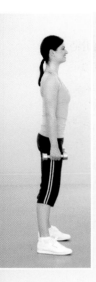

13 **Squat** Pick up two large free weights and stand with your feet parallel, shoulder width apart, knees soft. Hold the weights palms facing in. Shift your weight back onto your heels and as you inhale, bend your knees and reach back with your hips. Exhale and return to centre, tightening your buttocks as you straighten your legs. Repeat for 12 reps. **Do your next cardio interval, Steps 8–10.**

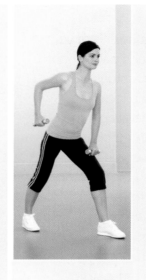

14 **Triceps kickback** Pick up two small free weights and stand in staggered lunge position, one foot back, leaning forwards. Bend the elbow on the same side to 90° and raise the upper arm as parallel to the floor as possible. Breathe in, then exhale as you extend the forearm behind you. Do 12 reps on each side. **Do your next cardio interval, Steps 8–10.**

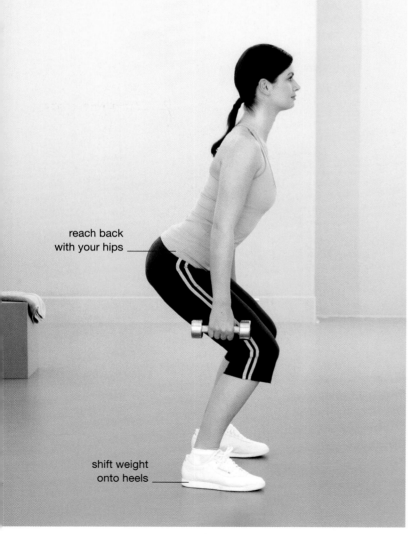

reach back with your hips ___

shift weight onto heels ___

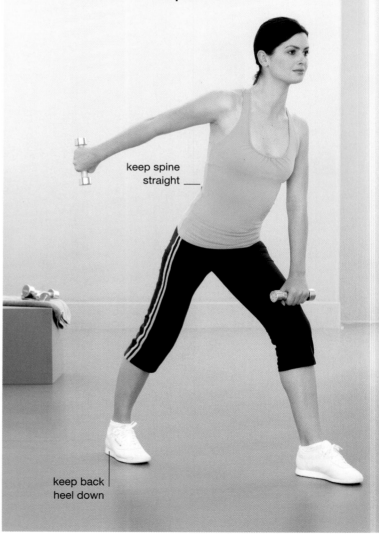

keep spine straight ___

keep back heel down

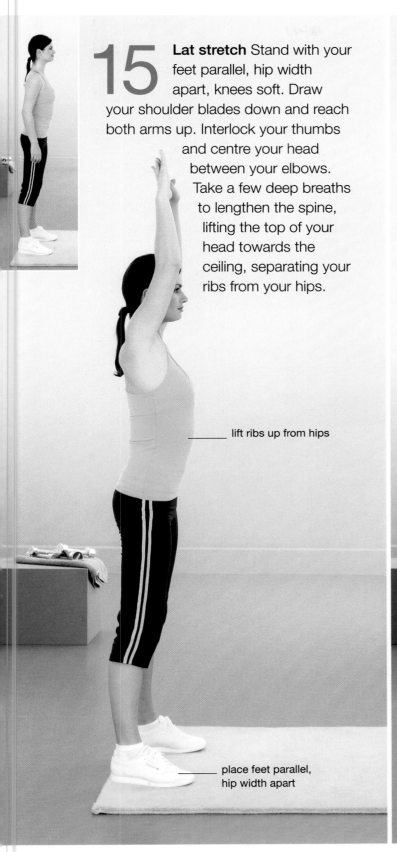

15 **Lat stretch** Stand with your feet parallel, hip width apart, knees soft. Draw your shoulder blades down and reach both arms up. Interlock your thumbs and centre your head between your elbows. Take a few deep breaths to lengthen the spine, lifting the top of your head towards the ceiling, separating your ribs from your hips.

lift ribs up from hips

place feet parallel, hip width apart

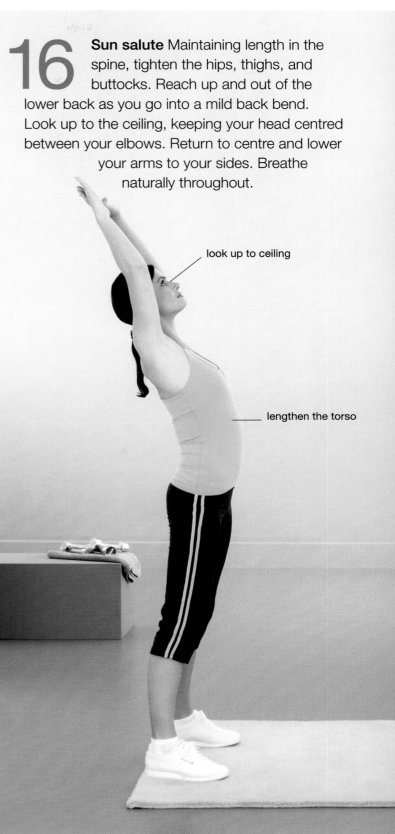

16 **Sun salute** Maintaining length in the spine, tighten the hips, thighs, and buttocks. Reach up and out of the lower back as you go into a mild back bend. Look up to the ceiling, keeping your head centred between your elbows. Return to centre and lower your arms to your sides. Breathe naturally throughout.

look up to ceiling

lengthen the torso

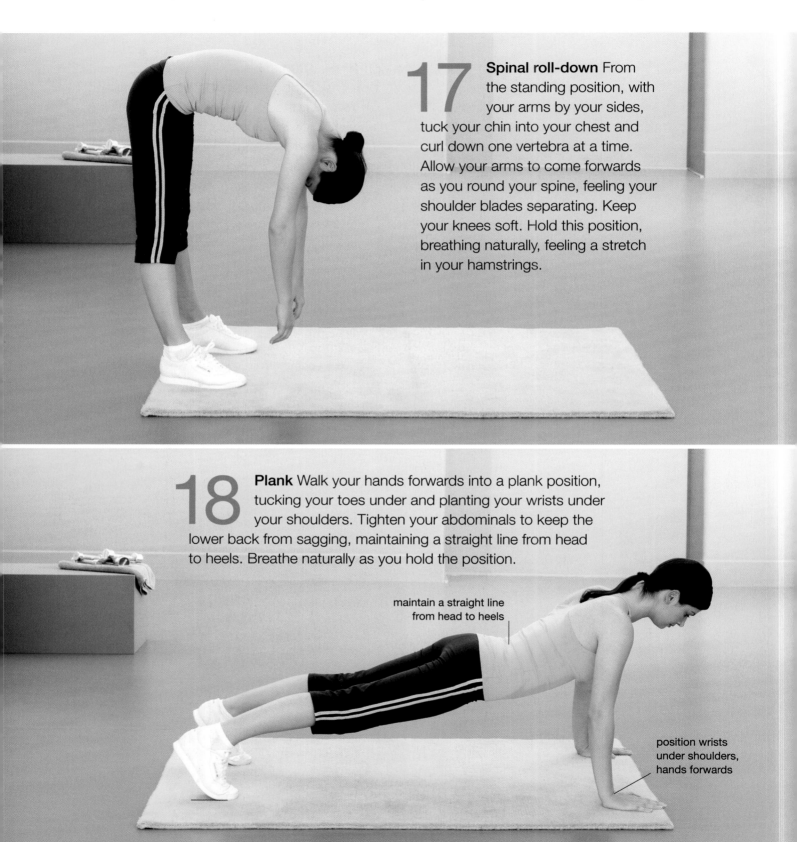

17 **Spinal roll-down** From the standing position, with your arms by your sides, tuck your chin into your chest and curl down one vertebra at a time. Allow your arms to come forwards as you round your spine, feeling your shoulder blades separating. Keep your knees soft. Hold this position, breathing naturally, feeling a stretch in your hamstrings.

18 **Plank** Walk your hands forwards into a plank position, tucking your toes under and planting your wrists under your shoulders. Tighten your abdominals to keep the lower back from sagging, maintaining a straight line from head to heels. Breathe naturally as you hold the position.

maintain a straight line from head to heels

position wrists under shoulders, hands forwards

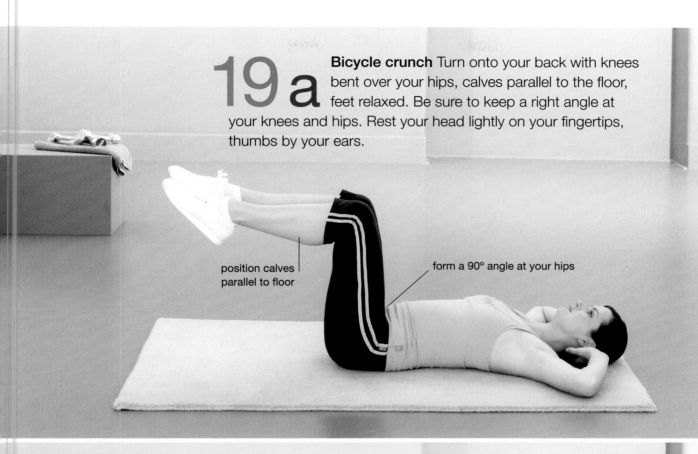

19 a

Bicycle crunch Turn onto your back with knees bent over your hips, calves parallel to the floor, feet relaxed. Be sure to keep a right angle at your knees and hips. Rest your head lightly on your fingertips, thumbs by your ears.

position calves parallel to floor

form a 90° angle at your hips

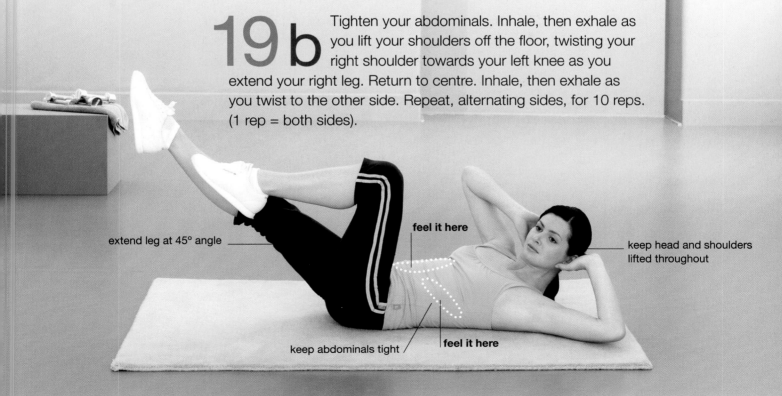

19 b

Tighten your abdominals. Inhale, then exhale as you lift your shoulders off the floor, twisting your right shoulder towards your left knee as you extend your right leg. Return to centre. Inhale, then exhale as you twist to the other side. Repeat, alternating sides, for 10 reps. (1 rep = both sides).

extend leg at 45° angle

feel it here

keep head and shoulders lifted throughout

keep abdominals tight

feel it here

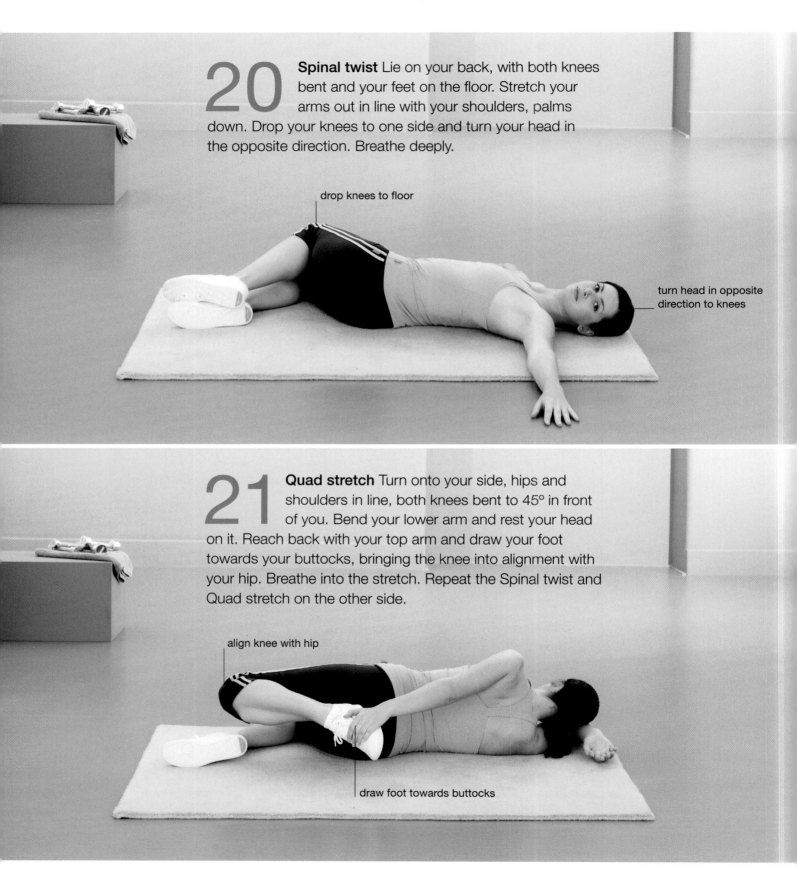

20 **Spinal twist** Lie on your back, with both knees bent and your feet on the floor. Stretch your arms out in line with your shoulders, palms down. Drop your knees to one side and turn your head in the opposite direction. Breathe deeply.

drop knees to floor

turn head in opposite direction to knees

21 **Quad stretch** Turn onto your side, hips and shoulders in line, both knees bent to 45° in front of you. Bend your lower arm and rest your head on it. Reach back with your top arm and draw your foot towards your buttocks, bringing the knee into alignment with your hip. Breathe into the stretch. Repeat the Spinal twist and Quad stretch on the other side.

align knee with hip

draw foot towards buttocks

22 **Sphinx** Roll onto your front. Bend your elbows and rest your forearms on the mat. Draw your shoulder blades down as you lift your chest, sliding your elbows forwards to be directly under your shoulders. Turn your head to one side, then the other, to stretch the neck. Hold each position and breathe naturally throughout.

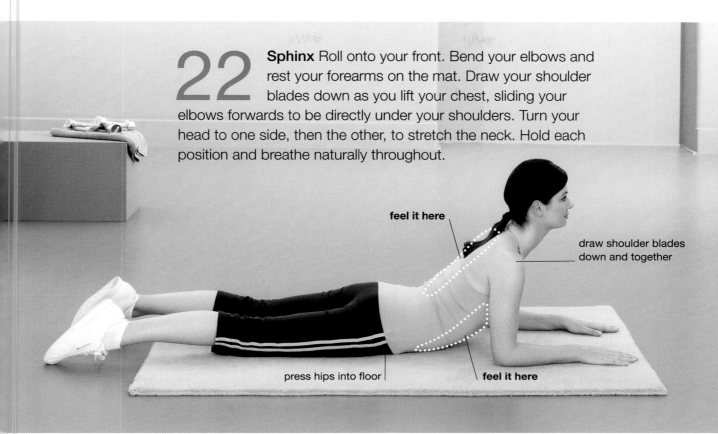

feel it here

draw shoulder blades down and together

press hips into floor

feel it here

23 **Child's pose** Sit back on your heels and bend forwards, forehead reaching to mat, arms stretching centre. Walk your hands to one side, keeping your head centred between your elbows, then stretch to the other side. With every exhale, let your body sink deeper into the position.

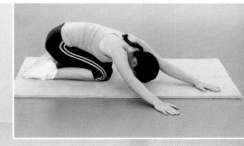

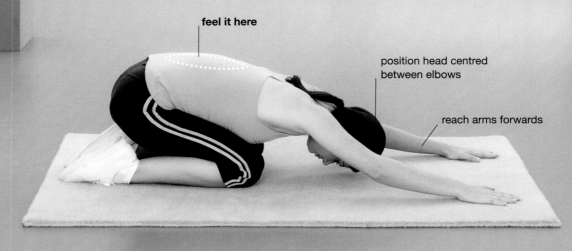

feel it here

position head centred between elbows

reach arms forwards

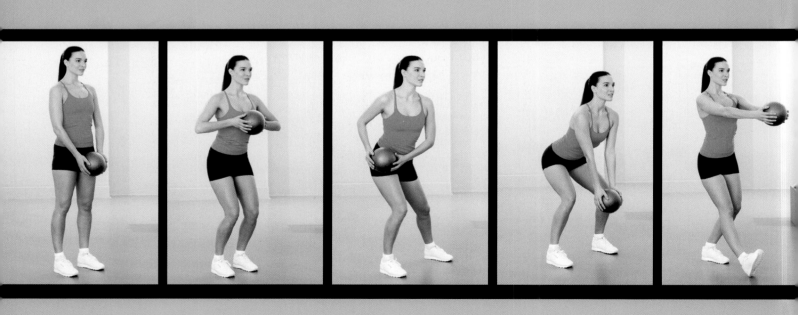

▶▶▶

building stamina

beach ball
workout

Improve your coordination and
balance while adding variety
to your workout with a ball

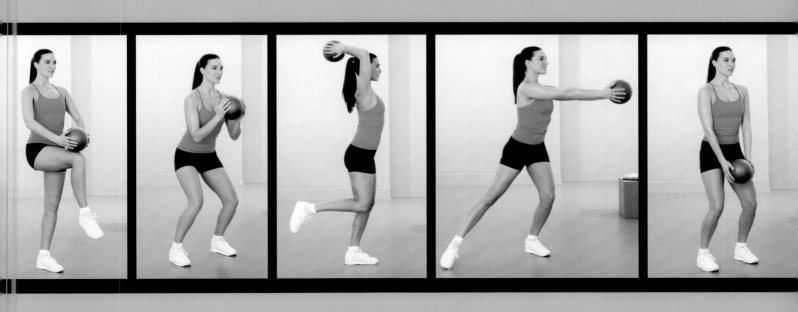

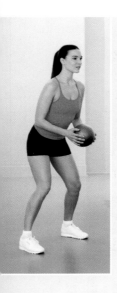

1 **Rock lunge** Stand with your feet parallel, slightly wider than shoulder width apart, knees bent. Lean forwards slightly and hold the ball in front of your hips. Straighten one leg and lunge the other way, moving the ball to your opposite hip. Repeat, alternating sides for a total of 8 reps (1 rep = both sides).

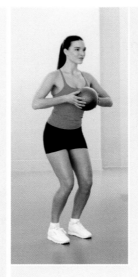

2 **Skater** Stand with your feet parallel, hip width apart, knees bent. Hold the ball in front of your chest. Keep one knee bent and shift your weight onto it as you extend the other leg out to the side, toe resting lightly on the floor. Stretch your arms out diagonally, pressing the ball away from your extended leg. Then return to the starting position and repeat, alternating sides, for a total of 8 reps (1 rep = both sides).

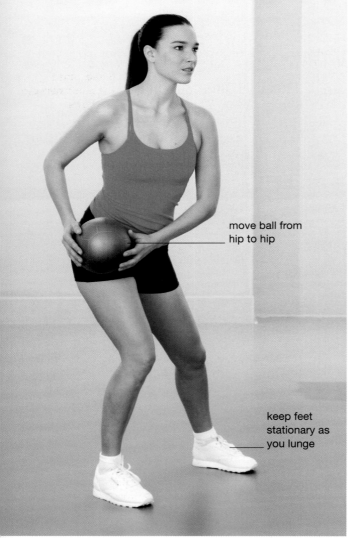

move ball from hip to hip

keep feet stationary as you lunge

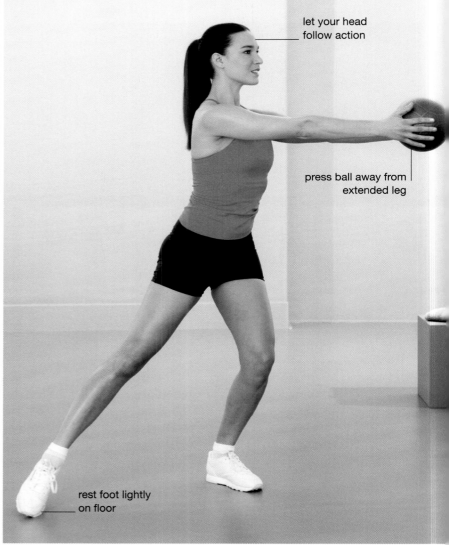

let your head follow action

press ball away from extended leg

rest foot lightly on floor

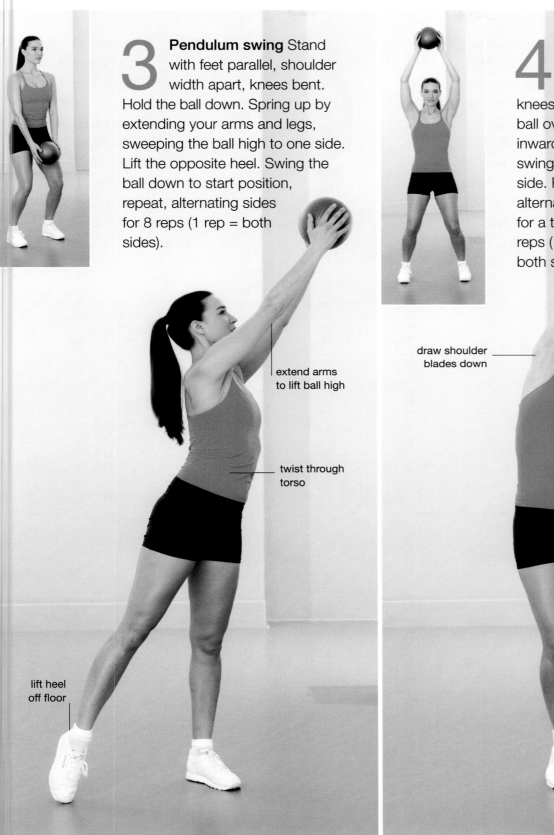

3 **Pendulum swing** Stand with feet parallel, shoulder width apart, knees bent. Hold the ball down. Spring up by extending your arms and legs, sweeping the ball high to one side. Lift the opposite heel. Swing the ball down to start position, repeat, alternating sides for 8 reps (1 rep = both sides).

extend arms to lift ball high

twist through torso

lift heel off floor

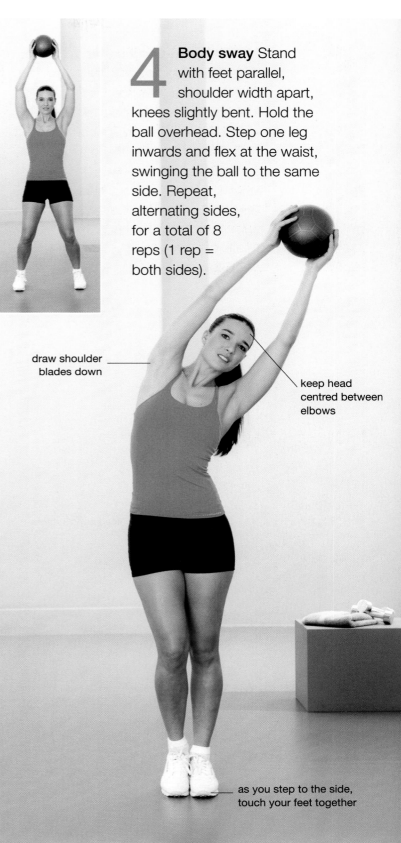

4 **Body sway** Stand with feet parallel, shoulder width apart, knees slightly bent. Hold the ball overhead. Step one leg inwards and flex at the waist, swinging the ball to the same side. Repeat, alternating sides, for a total of 8 reps (1 rep = both sides).

draw shoulder blades down

keep head centred between elbows

as you step to the side, touch your feet together

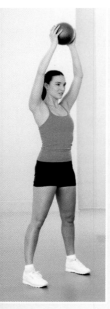

5 **Wood-chop squat** Still holding the ball above your head, stand with your feet parallel, shoulder width apart, knees soft. Bend your knees into a squat, reaching back with your hips, keeping your heels pressed into the floor. With your arms straight, "chop" the ball down, lowering it to the knees. Repeat 8 times.

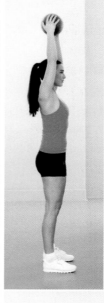

6 **Curl & press** Reach the ball towards the ceiling, then bend both elbows, lowering it behind your head. At the same time, bend one leg back, lifting your heel towards the buttocks. Repeat, alternating legs, for a total of 8 reps (1 rep = both sides). **Repeat Steps 5–1 (reverse order) to complete your warm up.**

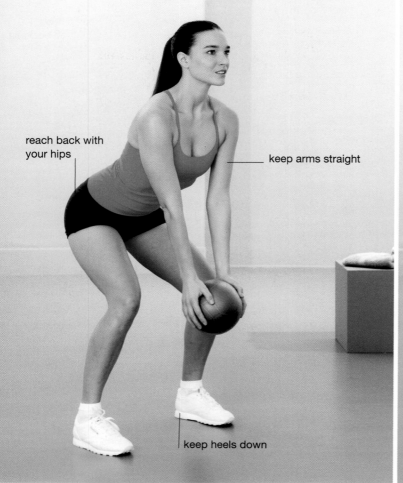

reach back with your hips

keep arms straight

keep heels down

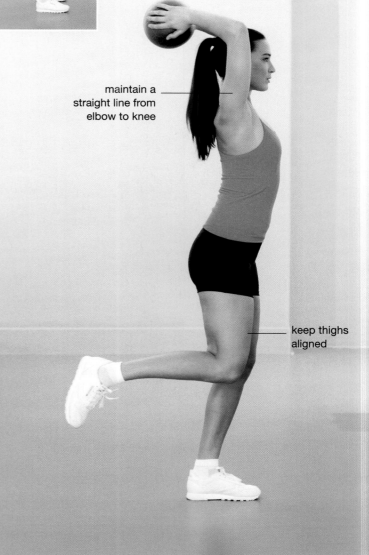

maintain a straight line from elbow to knee

keep thighs aligned

7a **Plié with front raise** Put down the ball and pick up one large weight for the first resistance exercise. Stand with your feet slightly wider than shoulder width apart, shift your weight to your heels, and turn your legs out from the hips until your feet are at 45° angles. Hold the weight horizontally with one hand at each end, your arms straight down in front.

7b As you inhale, bend your knees until your thighs are as parallel to the floor as possible; simultaneously lift the weight to shoulder height, keeping your arms straight. Exhale, press through your heels, and tighten your inner and outer thighs as you return to the starting position. Repeat 12 times.

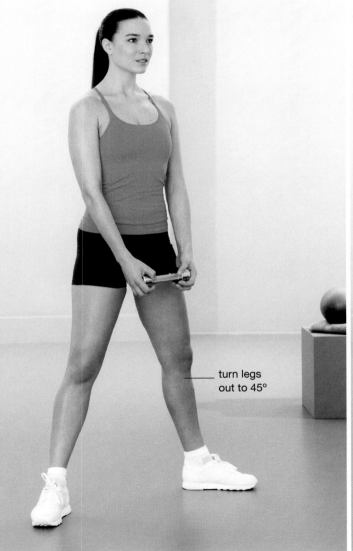

turn legs
out to 45°

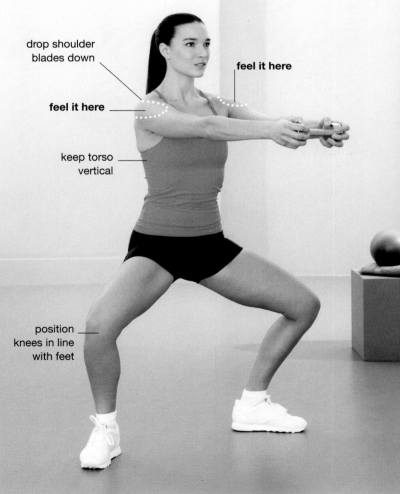

drop shoulder
blades down

feel it here

feel it here

keep torso
vertical

position
knees in line
with feet

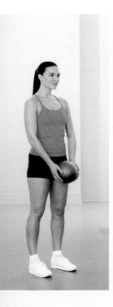

8 **Step & dig** Start your first cardio interval. Stand with your feet hip width apart, knees soft, feet parallel or slightly turned out. Hold the ball with your arms straight down. Tap your heel to the front, pointing your toes to the ceiling, as you bring the ball up to shoulder height. Keep your arms straight, not stiff. Alternate legs for a total of 8 reps (1 rep = both sides). Breathe naturally.

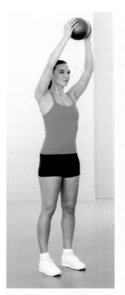

9 **Knee lift** Stand with your feet parallel, hip width apart, knees slightly bent. Hold the ball above your head, with elbows slightly rounded. Bring your knee up to hip height as you lower the ball towards your knee. Repeat, alternating legs for 8 reps (1 rep = both sides). Breathe naturally throughout.

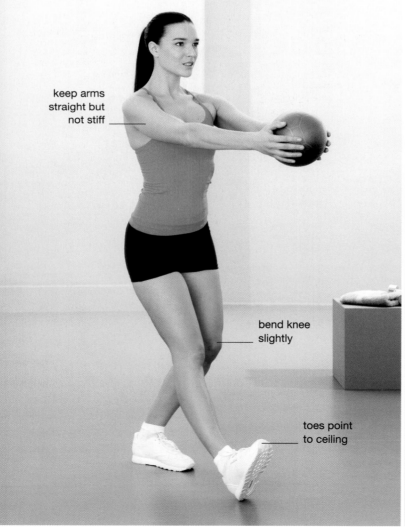

keep arms straight but not stiff

bend knee slightly

toes point to ceiling

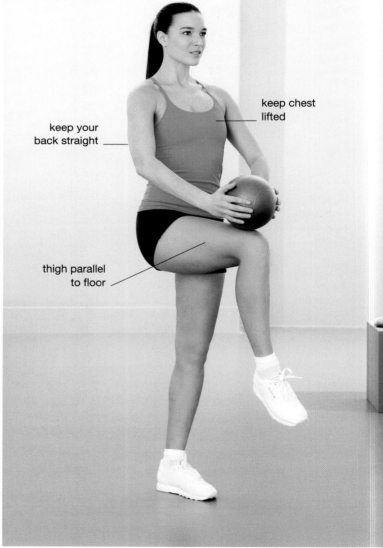

keep chest lifted

keep your back straight

thigh parallel to floor

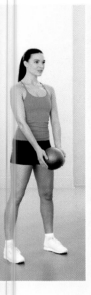

10a

Squat plus
Stand with your feet shoulder width apart, holding the ball with your arms straight down. Bend your knees into a squat, at the same time bending your elbows to lift the ball to your chest. Keep your weight centred, heels down. Reach back with your hips, keeping your knees behind your toes.

10b

Lift the ball up above your head as you straighten your legs. Then bend into the squat, ball to chest (10a), before returning to the starting position. Take full, deep breaths. Repeat the sequence 12 times. **Steps 8–10 complete the cardio interval.**

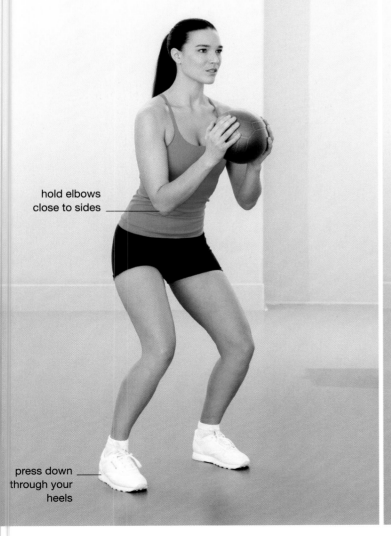

hold elbows close to sides

press down through your heels

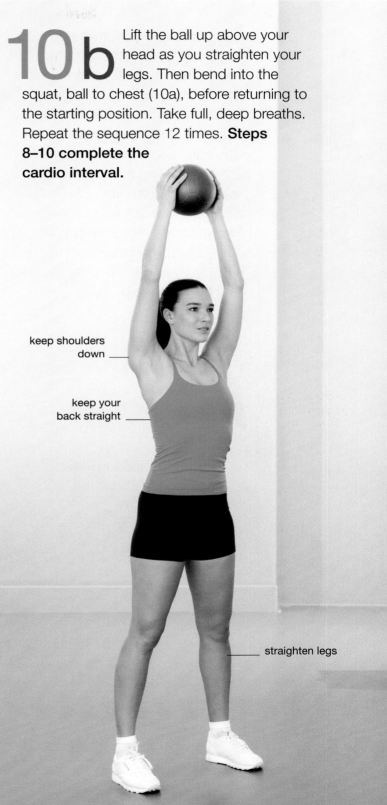

keep shoulders down

keep your back straight

straighten legs

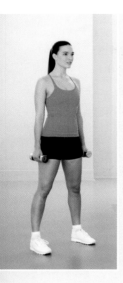

11a Squat with knee lift
Put down the beach ball and pick up two large free weights. Stand with your feet parallel, shoulder width apart, knees soft. Hold one weight in each hand, with your arms by your sides and palms facing in. Inhale as you squat: shift your weight back into your heels, reaching back with your hips and letting your torso lean forwards. Release your pelvis to allow a natural curve in your back.

11b
Exhale and straighten your legs. Shift your weight to one side and bring the other knee up to hip height. Balance for a moment, then return to the starting position (see inset, left). Squat again (see left), straighten your legs, and change sides for the knee lift (as shown below). Keep your hips level, chest lifted, eyes forwards throughout. Repeat for a total of 8 reps (1 rep = both sides). **Do your next cardio interval, Steps 8–10.**

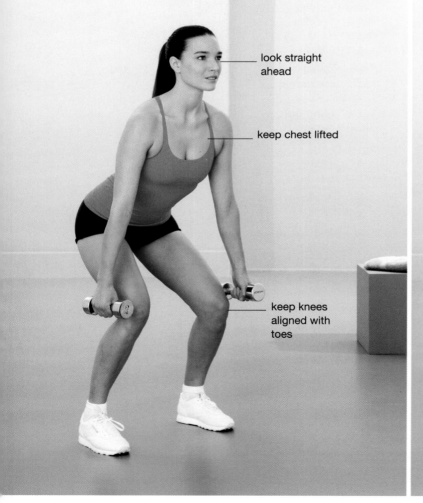

look straight ahead

keep chest lifted

keep knees aligned with toes

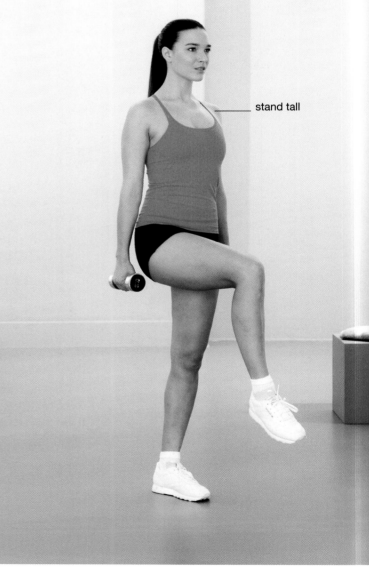

stand tall

12 a
Lunge & row
Exchange the ball for two large free weights. Stand with your feet parallel, hip width apart, knees soft. Hold the weights at your hips, palms in, elbows bent at right angles and close to your sides. Stabilize your shoulder blades by drawing them down and together. Keep your wrists straight, in line with your forearms.

12 b
Inhale as you step forwards with one leg, bending both knees. At the same time, straighten your arms, lowering the weights towards your knee. Exhale as you spring back, pulling the weights to your hips. Alternate legs for 8 reps (1 rep = both sides).
Do the next cardio interval, Steps 8–10.

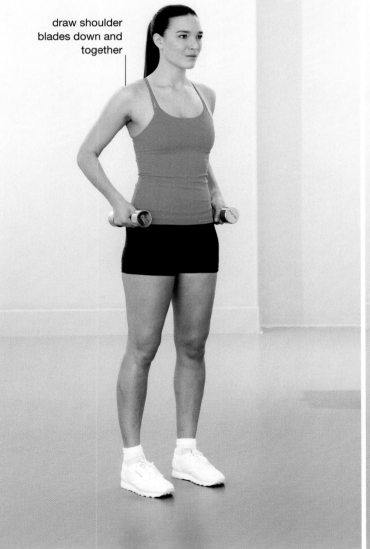

draw shoulder blades down and together

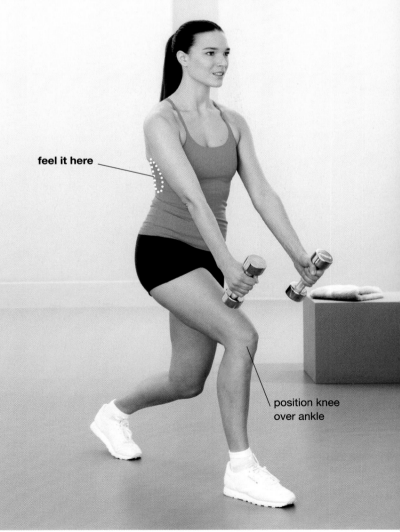

feel it here

position knee over ankle

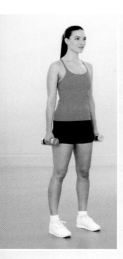

13a **Squat with weight shift**

Pick up two large weights. Stand with your feet parallel, hip width apart. Hold the weights by your sides. Shifting your weight into your heels, inhale as you bend your knees into a squat; at the same time, bend your elbows, bringing the weights up towards your shoulders.

13b

Exhale as you straighten your arms and legs to the starting position. Inhale again, then exhale as you shift your weight onto the balls of your feet and lift your heels high. Balance for a moment before lowering the heels onto the floor and preparing for the next squat. Do 8 reps, combining both moves. **Then do your next cardio interval, Steps 8–10.**

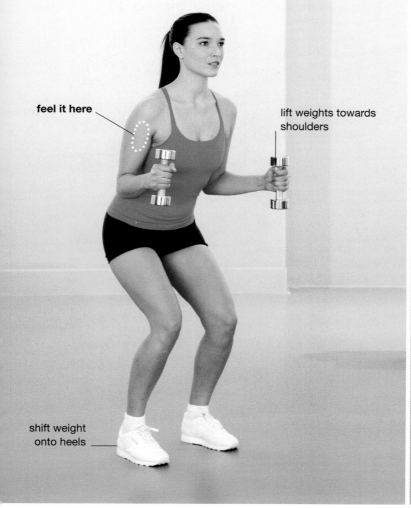

feel it here

lift weights towards shoulders

shift weight onto heels

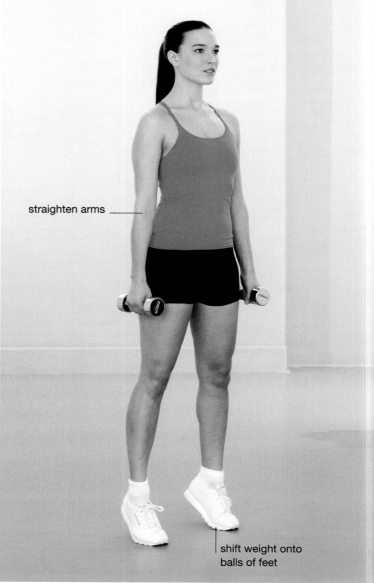

straighten arms

shift weight onto balls of feet

▶▶▶ **resistance** reverse fly/ triceps kickback

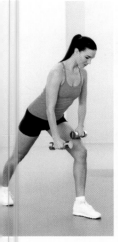

14 Reverse fly

Exchange the ball for two large free weights. Stand in staggered lunge position, one foot forwards and the arm on the same side resting on your thigh. Draw your shoulder blade in and exhale as you lift the other arm out to the side at shoulder height. Repeat 12 times, then switch sides. **Do your next cardio interval, Steps 8–10.**

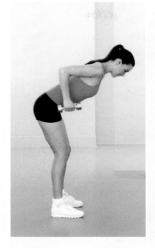

15 Triceps kickback

Exchange the ball for two large weights. Bend your knees and hinge forwards. Bend your elbows to 90° and raise your upper arms parallel to the floor. Exhale, extending forearms behind. Inhale as you bend your elbows. Repeat 12 times. **Do your next cardio interval, Steps 8–10.**

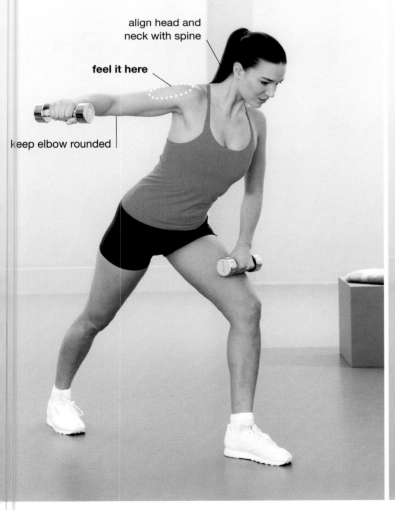

align head and neck with spine

feel it here

keep elbow rounded

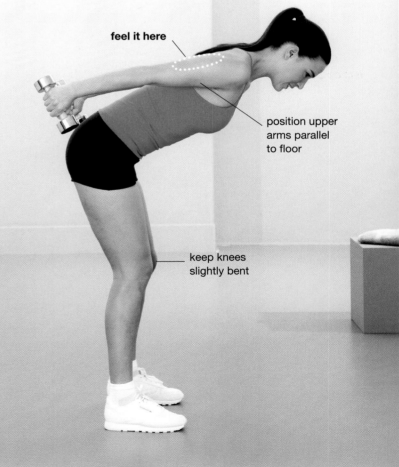

feel it here

position upper arms parallel to floor

keep knees slightly bent

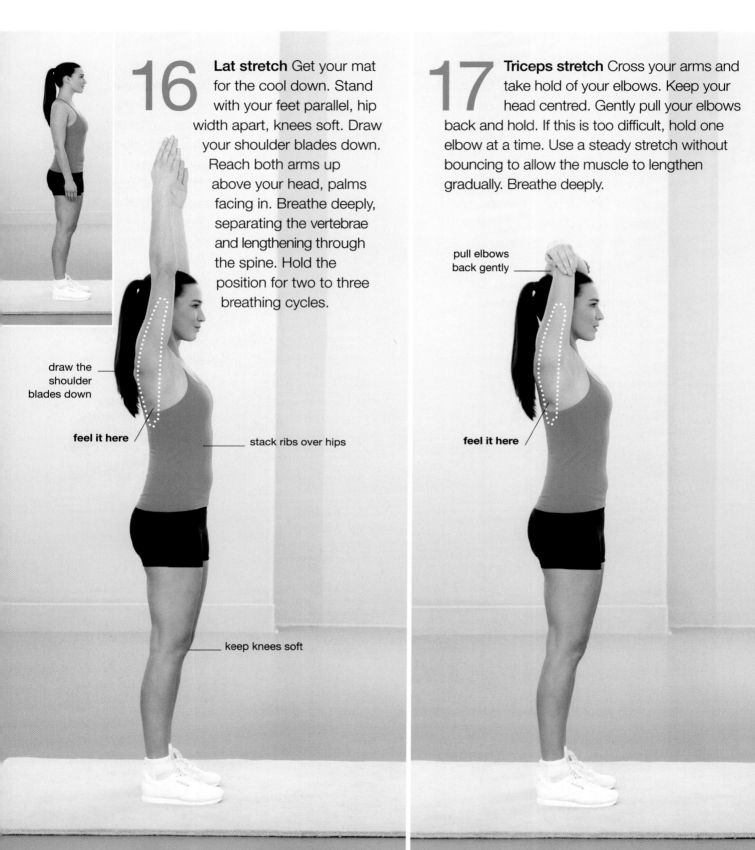

16 **Lat stretch** Get your mat for the cool down. Stand with your feet parallel, hip width apart, knees soft. Draw your shoulder blades down. Reach both arms up above your head, palms facing in. Breathe deeply, separating the vertebrae and lengthening through the spine. Hold the position for two to three breathing cycles.

draw the shoulder blades down

feel it here

stack ribs over hips

keep knees soft

17 **Triceps stretch** Cross your arms and take hold of your elbows. Keep your head centred. Gently pull your elbows back and hold. If this is too difficult, hold one elbow at a time. Use a steady stretch without bouncing to allow the muscle to lengthen gradually. Breathe deeply.

pull elbows back gently

feel it here

18 **Side bend** Still holding your elbows, and with your head centred, lift up from the waist and bend to one side, feeling a stretch all the way down your side to the hip. Hold, breathing into the stretch; then pass through the centre and bend to the other side. Hold, take a deep breath and then return to centre.

19 **Forward bend** From the centre position reach forward with your arms at shoulder height. Cross your wrists and turn your palms inwards to bring them together, thumbs facing down. Round your upper back, head and neck aligned with your spine, ears between your upper arms. Separate your shoulder blades and reach as far forward as possible. Breathe and relax deeper into the stretch with each exhalation.

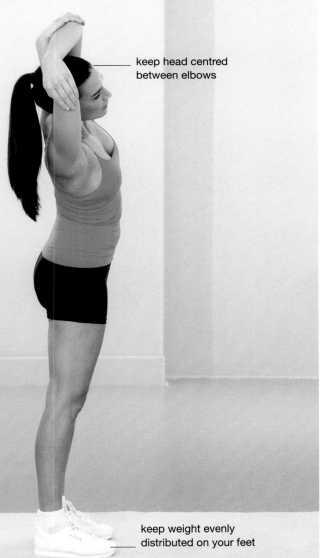

keep head centred between elbows

keep weight evenly distributed on your feet

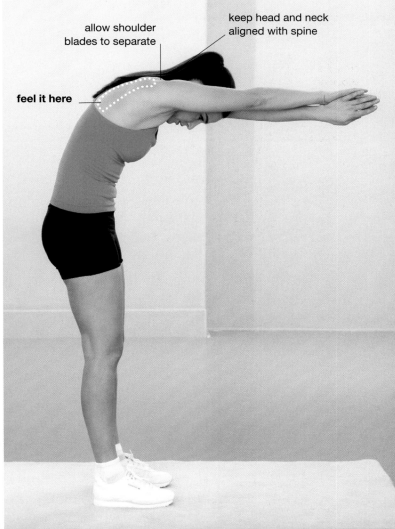

allow shoulder blades to separate

keep head and neck aligned with spine

feel it here

20 Spinal roll-down

From the Forward Bend Position, drop your arms to your sides, tuck your chin into your chest, and roll down through the spine, one vertebra at a time. Allow your arms to come forwards and the shoulder blades to separate.

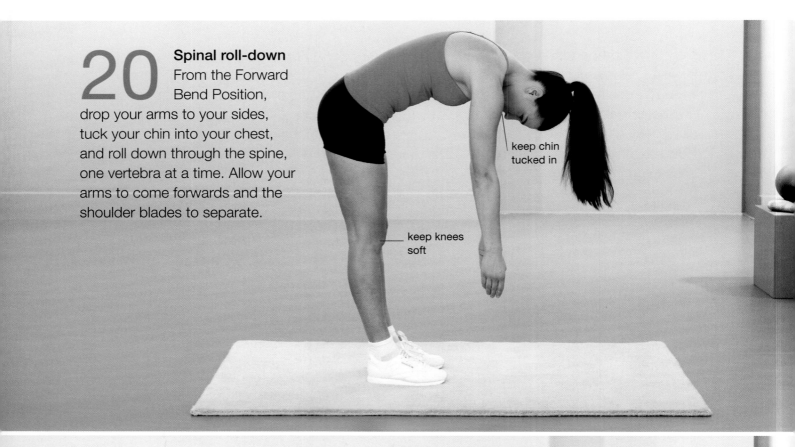

keep chin tucked in

keep knees soft

21 Downward dog

Bend down, place your palms on the mat and walk your hands forwards. Reach up with your hips and keep lengthening through the spine. Press your heels towards the floor. If necessary, bend your knees slightly to release your low back. Breathe and stretch.

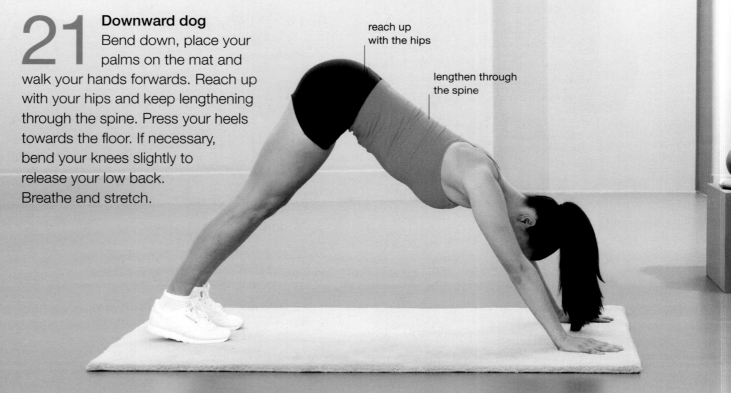

reach up with the hips

lengthen through the spine

22 **Plank** Walk forwards and place your forearms on the mat, elbows directly under your shoulders, palms facing in, hands in loose fists. Tighten your abdominal and back muscles to keep your torso lifted in a straight line from head to toe. Tuck your toes under slightly: you will feel a stretch in your calves. Hold the position, breathing naturally.

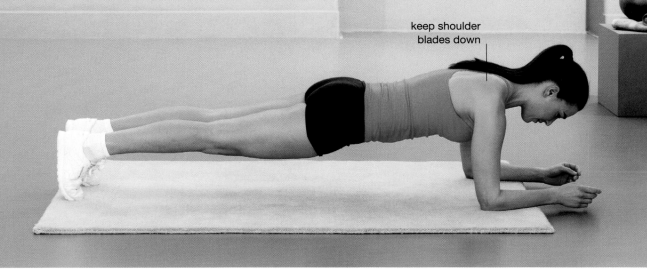

keep shoulder blades down

23 **Child's pose** Bend your knees and reach back with your hips until your buttocks rest on your heels. At the same time round forwards, curving the spine, forehead towards floor. Reach your arms to the front to stretch your lats, chest, and shoulders. With every exhale, sink deeper into the position; mind and body calm. Move back into the plank, bending your elbows and straightening your legs. Finally, repeat the Child's pose.

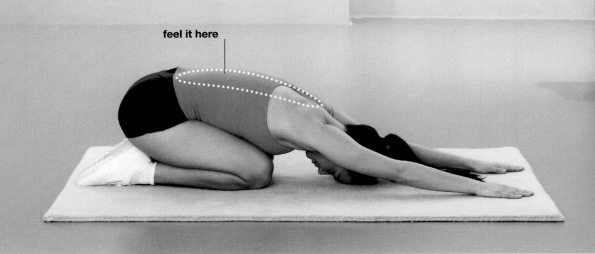

feel it here

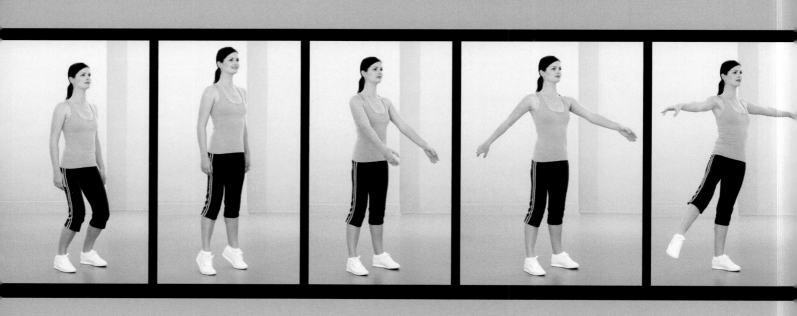

getting stronger

hop, jig, and jump workout

Experience the child-like joy of hopping
and jumping as you release endorphins
with this upbeat workout

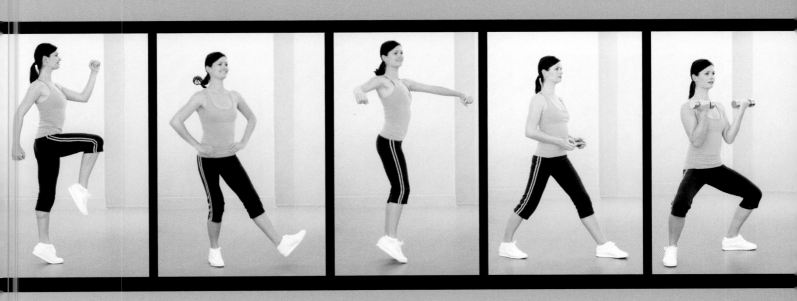

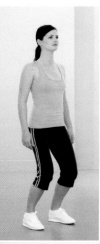

1 **Bend & raise** Stand with your feet parallel, hip width apart, knees soft, arms by your sides. Tighten your abdominals and lift your chest. Bend your knees (see inset) then straighten your legs. Shift your weight to the balls of your feet and lift your heels, resisting the floor. Continue bending and then rising up, allowing your arms to swing naturally forwards, for a total of 8 times.

2 **Double arm swing** Continue to bend your knees rhythmically as you swing your arms to back and front. From the starting position of bent knees (see inset), feet flat on the floor, straighten your legs and swing your arms behind. Bend your knees again as your arms pass through the centre and then swing them in front as you straighten your legs. Repeat for a total of 8 swings, back to front.

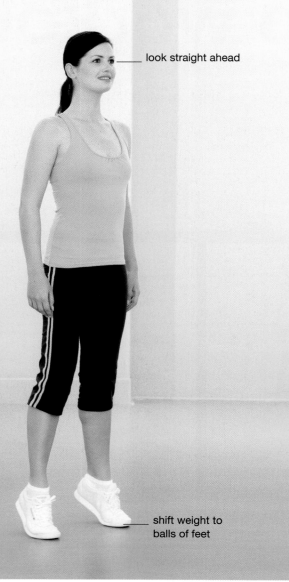

look straight ahead

shift weight to balls of feet

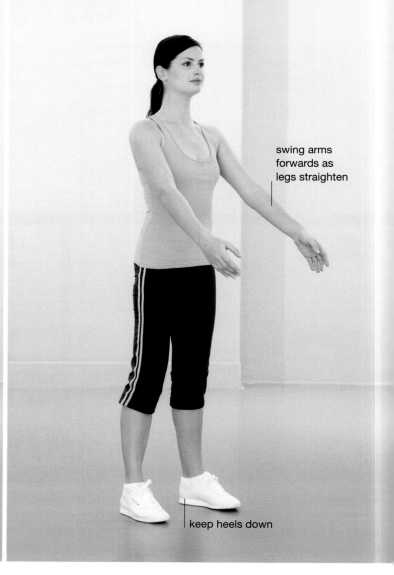

swing arms forwards as legs straighten

keep heels down

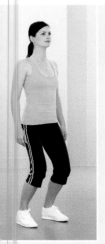

3 **Single arm swing** Continue to bend your knees rhythmically, but change the arms, swinging one forwards and the other back every time you straighten your legs. Keep your heels down, knees in line with toes. Keep your shoulder blades down as you swing your arms. Your chest stays lifted, chin level. Repeat, alternating arms, for a total of 8 reps (1 rep = both sides).

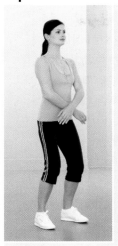

4 **Cross & open** Continuing with rhythmic knee bends, change your arms to cross in front as you bend your knees and then lift them out to the sides as you straighten your legs. Keep your shoulder blades down as you lift your arms to shoulder height, palms down. Bend and straighten, lifting your arms out to the sides,16 times.

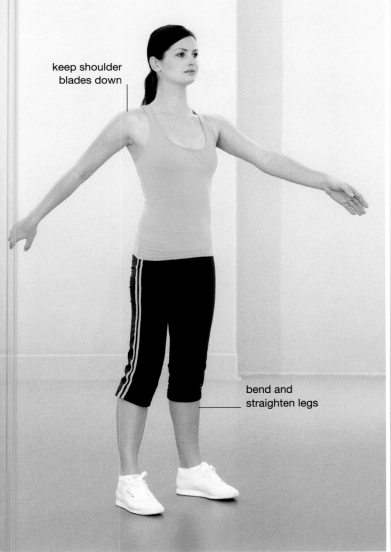

keep shoulder blades down

bend and straighten legs

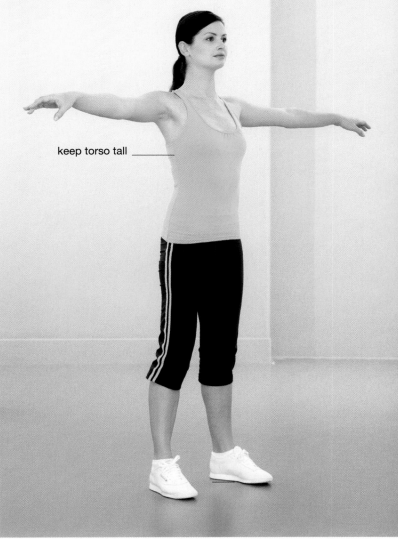

keep torso tall

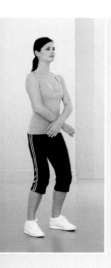

5 **Lateral lift** Arms stay the same as you bend and straighten your knees, but you add a side leg lift. Bend your knees as you cross your arms in front, then straighten both legs and lift one to the side as you raise your arms. Keep your hips level, shoulders down. Repeat, alternating legs, for a total of 8 reps (1 rep = both sides).

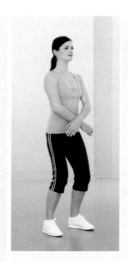

6 **Jumping jack** Continue to raise and lower your arms, but change your legs. As you cross your arms in front, jump your feet together. As you raise your arms to shoulder height, tap one foot out to the side. Alternate sides for 8 reps (1 rep = both sides). **Repeat Steps 5–1 (in reverse) to complete your warm up.**

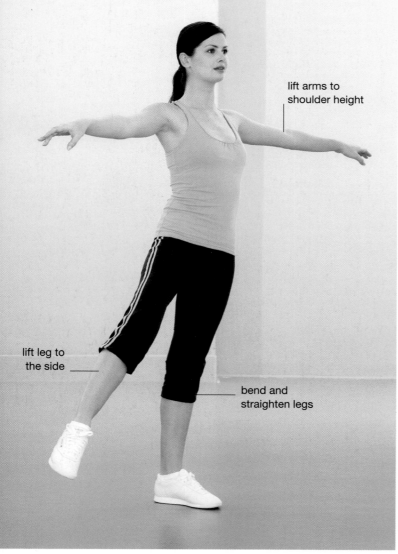

lift arms to shoulder height

lift leg to the side

bend and straighten legs

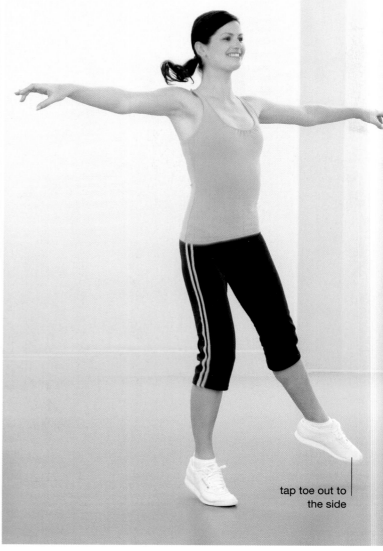

tap toe out to the side

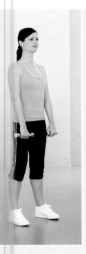

7a **Hip hinge & reverse fly** Pick up two small weights for your first resistance exercise. Stand up straight, feet parallel, hip width apart, shoulders down. Hold a weight in each hand in front of your thighs, palms facing back. Bend your knees as you hinge forwards from the hips, maintaining neutral spine alignment. The weights are now directly under your shoulders.

7b Inhale, then, as you exhale, raise your arms to the sides, in line with the shoulders, to shoulder height. Keep shoulder blades together as you lift your arms, elbows rounded, palms backwards. Inhale and lower your arms, then exhale as you straighten your hips and knees to return to start position (see inset). Repeat combination for 8 reps.

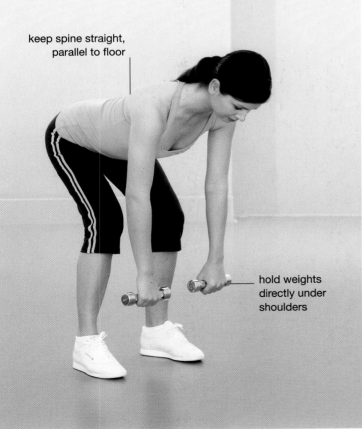

keep spine straight, parallel to floor

hold weights directly under shoulders

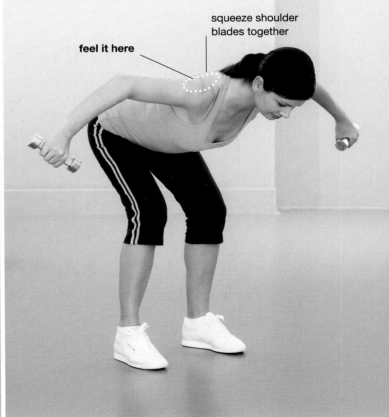

squeeze shoulder blades together

feel it here

8 **Step-hop** Put down the weights for the first cardio interval. Stand with your feet parallel, hip width apart, arms by your sides. Step forwards with one leg and hop on it, as your raise the other knee to hip height. The arm opposite the raised leg swings forwards, elbow bent. Lower the leg and step back to the starting position. Alternate legs, swinging your arms in opposition, for a total of 6 reps (1 rep = both sides).

9 **Jig** To begin, jump in place, feet hip width apart, hands on your hips. Hop on one leg, extending the other leg on a diagonal, digging your heel into the floor, toe pointing towards the ceiling. Bring the exended leg back and repeat on the other side. Keep your upper body vertical, chest lifted, eyes looking straight ahead. Alternate legs for a total of 8 reps (1 rep = both sides).

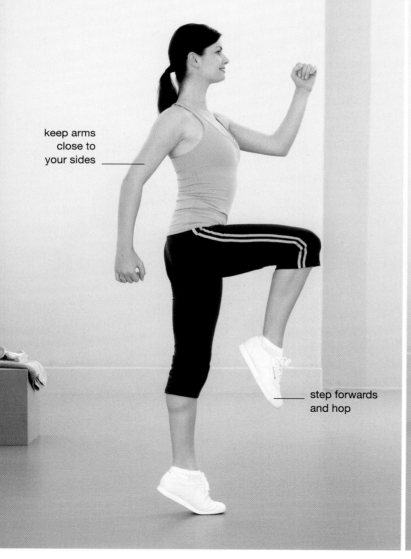

keep arms close to your sides

step forwards and hop

10 **Jump & twist** With your feet together, arms out to the sides, contract your abdominals and jump up, rotating your hips to one side. Turn your hips, knees, and feet as a unit. Land with your knees bent. Keep your torso upright, your shoulders facing forwards. Alternate sides for a total of 8 reps (1 rep = both sides). **Steps 8–10 complete your cardio interval, which you will repeat after each resistance exercise.**

11a **Lunge & twist** Pick up one large free weight. Step forwards with one leg into a staggered lunge position. Hold the weight with both hands horizontally in front of your waist, elbows bent. Keep your weight centred between your legs, your back heel down and your feet parallel. Your shoulders should be square to the front, your eyes looking straight ahead.

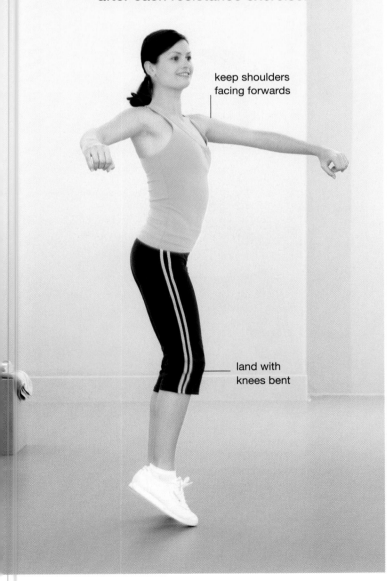

keep shoulders facing forwards

land with knees bent

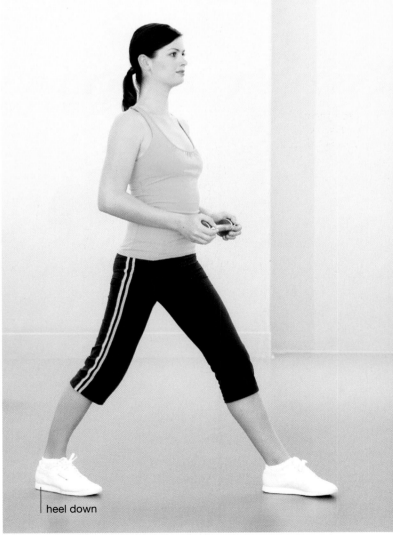

heel down

11b

Inhale as you bend both knees into a low lunge. Bend your front knee at a right angle directly over the ankle, the thigh parallel to the floor; bend your back knee close to the floor with the back heel lifted. As you come into the lunge, twist through your torso, reaching the weight towards your little toe. Keep your shoulder blades drawn together and your head and neck aligned with your spine, being careful not to round the upper back.

11c

Exhale as you return to the starting position and then lift the weight high on a diagonal above your opposite shoulder, elbows bent. Keep looking forwards. Do 6 reps of the sequence, bending your knees into a lunge as you lower the weight before lifting it again. Switch sides for another 6 reps. **Then do your next cardio interval, Steps 8–10.**

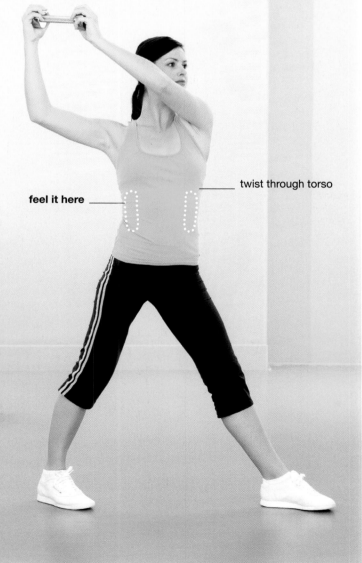

feel it here _____   twist through torso

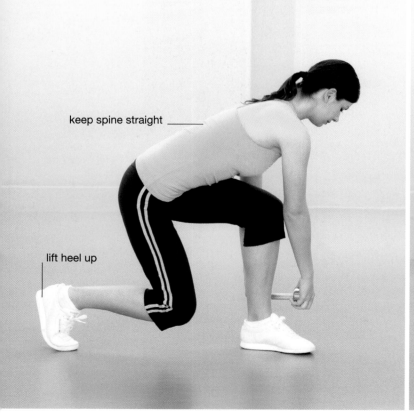

keep spine straight _____

lift heel up

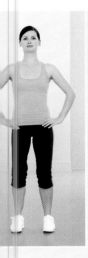

12 a

Side-squat, jump
Stand with your feet parallel, hip width apart, knees soft, your hands on your hips. Step one leg to the side so that your feet are shoulder width apart. Shift your weight back onto your heels as you bend your knees into a squat. Reach back with your hips, keeping your chest lifted.

12 b

Spring from both feet, jumping straight up. Land in a squat, knees bent, weight centred. Straighten your legs, step back to centre, and repeat, stepping to the other side. Do 4 reps (1 rep = both sides) for a total of 8 squats. **Do the next cardio interval, Steps 8–10.**

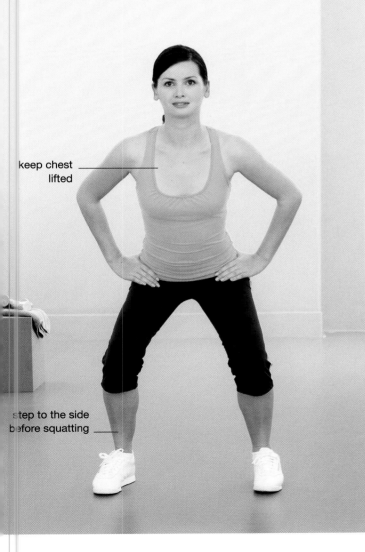

keep chest lifted

step to the side before squatting

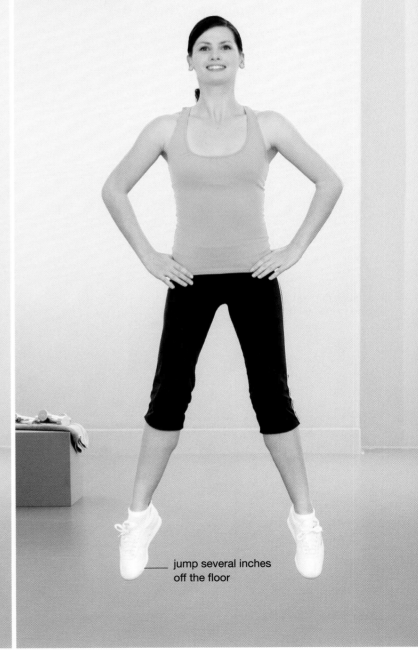

jump several inches off the floor

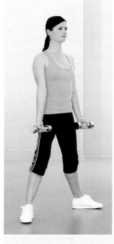

13 **Balance & press** Stand with feet parallel, hip width apart. Hold two small weights at shoulder height. Exhale, extending one arm, lifting opposite knee. Balance, inhale and step in place, alternating sides for 8 reps (1 rep = both sides). **Do your next cardio interval, Steps 8–10.**

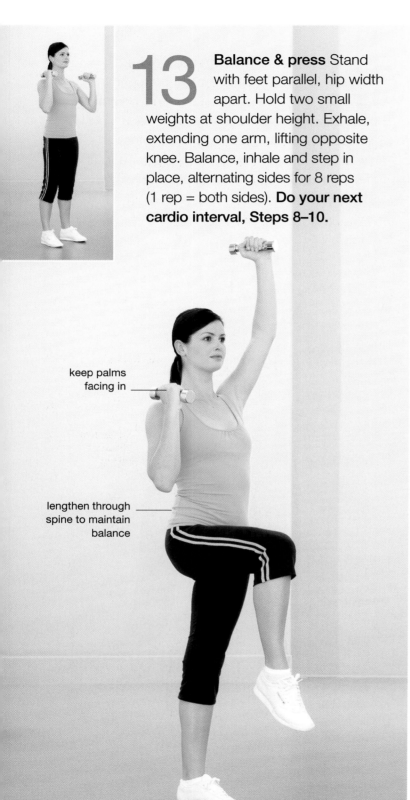

keep palms facing in

lengthen through spine to maintain balance

14 **Plié & curl** Pick up two large weights, holding one in each hand. Stand in a wide stance, legs turned out to 45°. Keep your arms by your sides. Inhale and bend your knees and elbows at the same time, lifting the weights towards your shoulders. Exhale as you straighten your arms and legs. **Do your next cardio interval, Steps 8–10.**

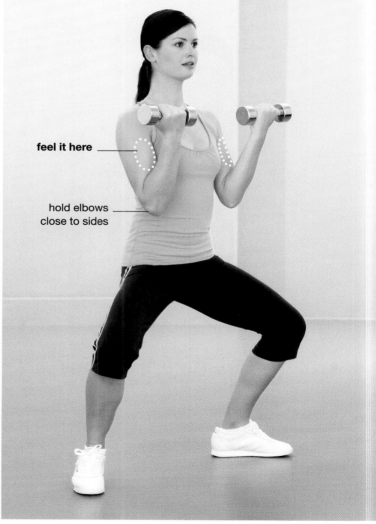

feel it here

hold elbows close to sides

15a
Lateral lift Pick up two small weights. Stand with your feet parallel, hip width apart, knees bent. Hold one weight in each hand, arms by your sides, palms facing inwards. Make sure your torso is aligned and ready for action: stack your ribs over your hips, engage the abdominals, draw your shoulder blades down, and lift your chest.

15b
Inhale, then exhale as you straighten your legs, lifting one to the side, as you raise both arms to shoulder height, palms down. Your arms should be straight but not stiff. Inhale, then return to the starting position, bending the knees and squaring the hips. Alternate legs, lifting both arms every time for 12 reps (1 rep = both sides).

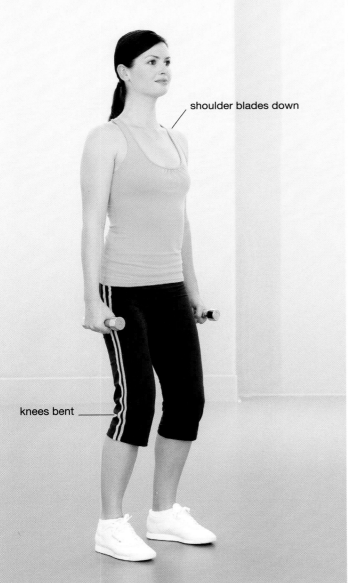

shoulder blades down

knees bent

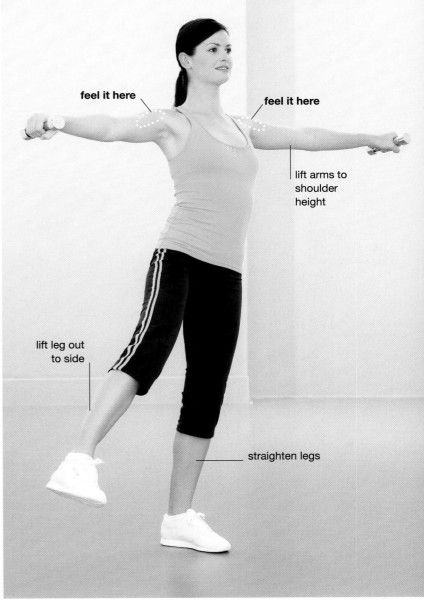

feel it here

feel it here

lift arms to shoulder height

lift leg out to side

straighten legs

16 **Flat back stretch** Get your mat for the cool down, and stand with your legs hip width apart, hands on your hips. Lengthen through the spine, lifting the top of your head towards the ceiling. Draw your shoulder blades down and together. Bend forwards from your hips until your back is parallel to the floor, still elongating the spine by reaching your head forwards. Keep your knees straight, but not locked. Breathe deeply while you hold the stretch.

17 **Spinal twist** From the flat back position, reach one hand across your body to the opposite foot, and lift the other arm straight up to the ceiling, palm forwards. If you are able, press the heel of the supporting hand down on the mat. However, you may be more comfortable resting it on your ankle. Keep your knees straight and your hips level. Breathe naturally throughout, then swap sides and repeat.

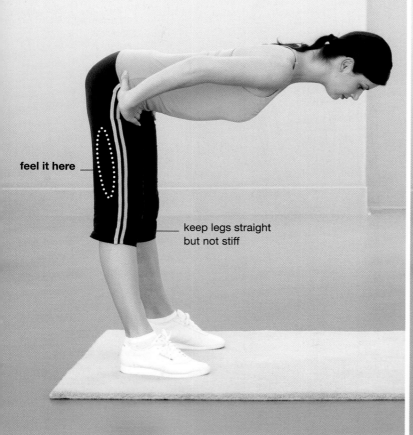

feel it here

keep legs straight but not stiff

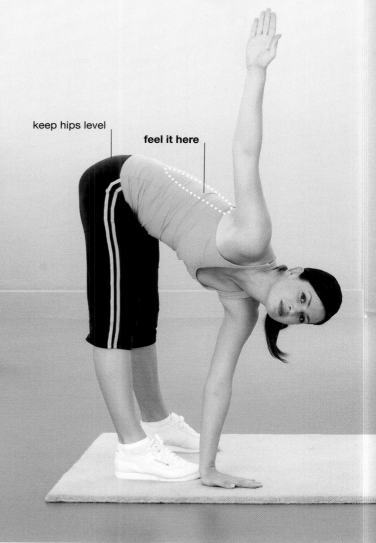

keep hips level

feel it here

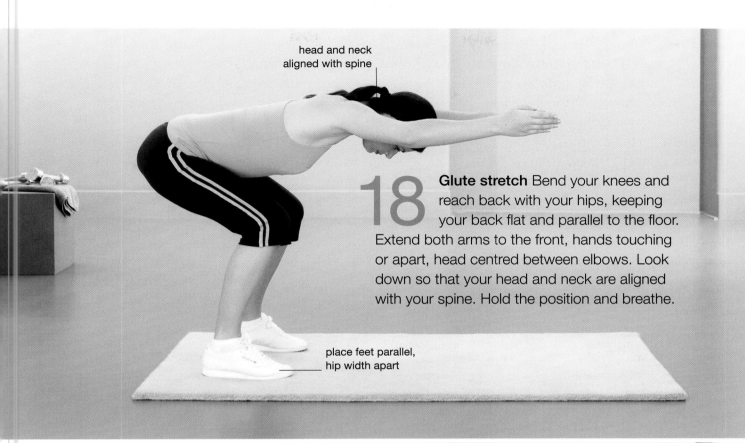

head and neck
aligned with spine

18 **Glute stretch** Bend your knees and reach back with your hips, keeping your back flat and parallel to the floor. Extend both arms to the front, hands touching or apart, head centred between elbows. Look down so that your head and neck are aligned with your spine. Hold the position and breathe.

place feet parallel,
hip width apart

19 **Arm and leg lift** Kneel on all fours, wrists beneath shoulders, knees under hips. Lift one leg to the back, keeping the knee straight, then reach forwards with the opposite hand. Use deep breathing to increase the stretch, reaching further on every exhale.

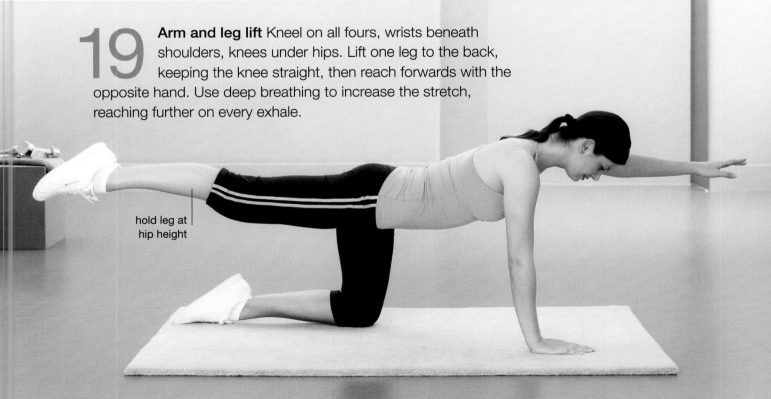

hold leg at
hip height

20 **Calf stretch** Keep your arms planted and extend one leg behind you, placing your toes on the floor and pressing the heel back. Breathe naturally as you stretch, then swap legs.

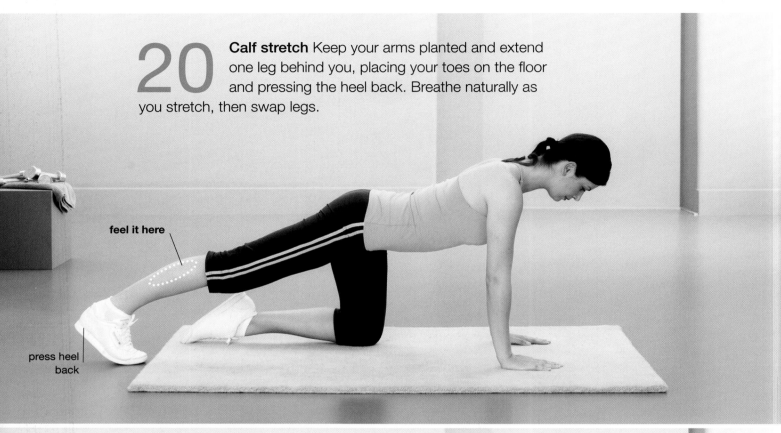

feel it here

press heel back

21 **Spinal curve** Kneel on all fours, knees under your hips, hip width apart. Position your wrists under your shoulders. Lift your head and your hips up, curving the spine into a "C" shape. Alternate this with the Spinal arch on the opposite page, repeating 3 times in all.

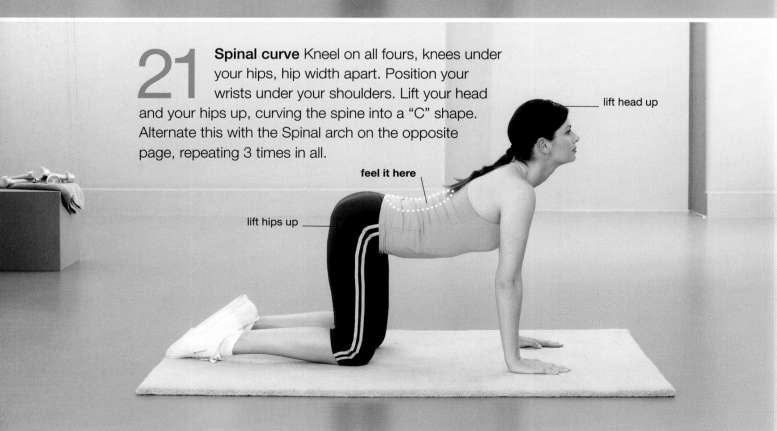

lift head up

feel it here

lift hips up

22 **Spinal arch** Start from a kneeling positon, knees under hips, wrists under shoulders, your back neutral. Then arch your spine, rounding it up to the ceiling by tucking your hips under and dropping your head between your arms. Alternate this with Spinal curve (opposite page), repeating 3 times in all.

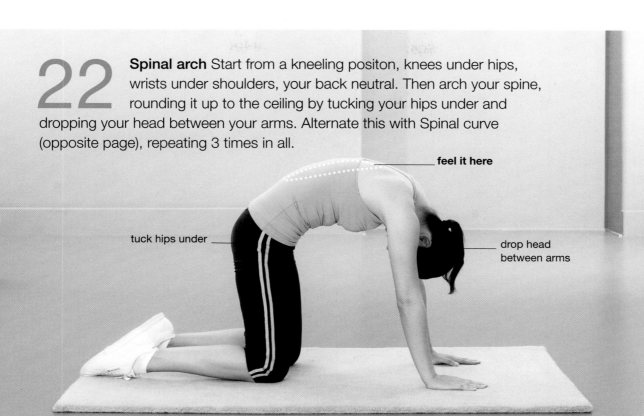

feel it here

tuck hips under

drop head between arms

23 **Child's pose** Sit back, reaching your hips towards your heels, at the same time rounding forward and extending your arms in front of you until your head rests on the mat. Keep your elbows off the mat to get the best stretch. Sink down into the position, holding for 3 deep breathing cycles, and sinking deeper into the position with each exhalation.

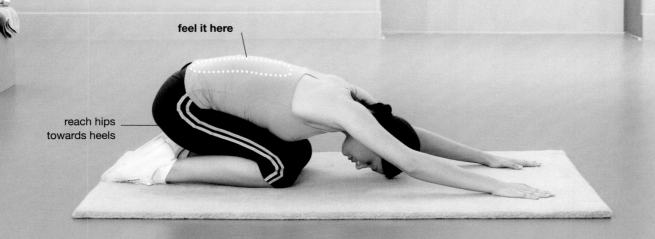

feel it here

reach hips towards heels

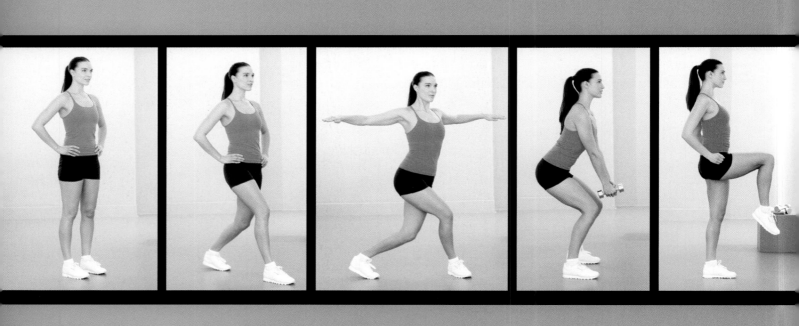

get fit plus

lunge around the clock workout

Challenge yourself with more
complex moves to advance
your skills and fitness levels

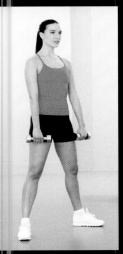
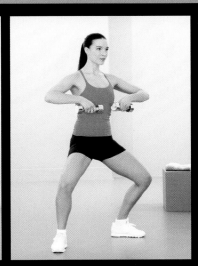
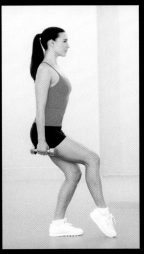
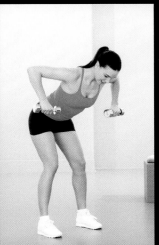
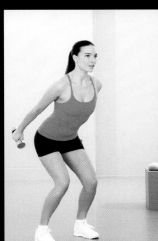

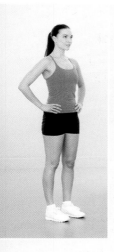

1 **Front lunge** Stand with feet parallel, hip width apart, knees soft, hands on hips. Inhale as you step forwards, bending knees slightly. Then exhale and push off with your front leg to spring back to the centre. Alternate sides for 8 reps (1 rep = both sides).

2 **Opposite arm raise** Continue to lunge, alternating legs, and add your arms. From the starting position, feet parallel, hip width apart, step forwards, bending your knees a little deeper, lifting your back heel and always keeping your knee over the ankle. At the same time, raise your hands to shoulder height, palms in, the opposite arm to the front and the other one behind. Keep your torso upright, chest lifted, chin level. Alternate legs and arms for 8 reps (1 rep = both sides).

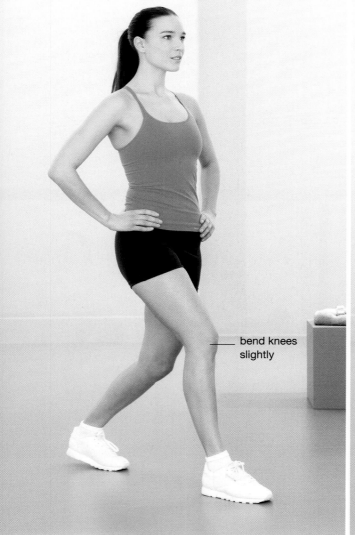

bend knees slightly

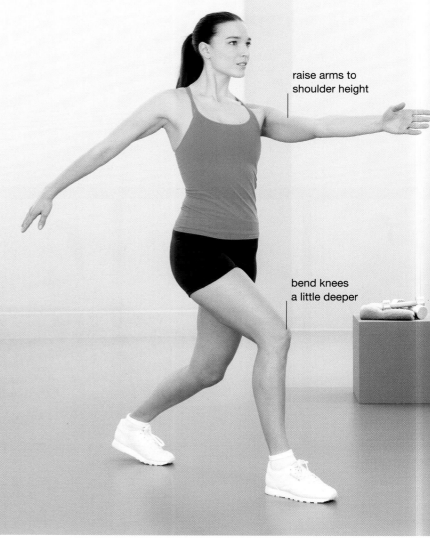

raise arms to shoulder height

bend knees a little deeper

3 **Arm reach** Continue to lunge, but now raise both arms to the front, lifting as you lunge, and increasing the bend in your knees. Pull your shoulder blades down and together to stabilize them as you extend your arms forwards. Lower your arms to your sides as you return to centre. Continue, alternating legs, for 8 reps (1 rep = both sides).

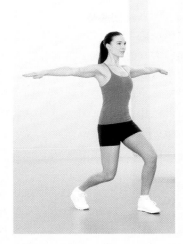

4 **Diagonal lunge** From the centre, pivot on the back foot and step out to 11 o'clock, lifting your arms to the sides. Spring back to centre, lowering your arms, then lunge out on the opposite diagonal to 1 o'clock. Repeat for 8 reps.

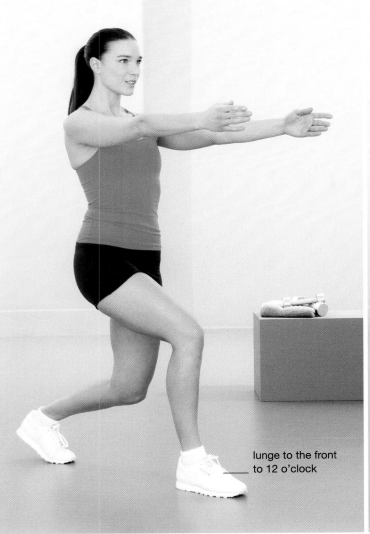

lunge to the front to 12 o'clock

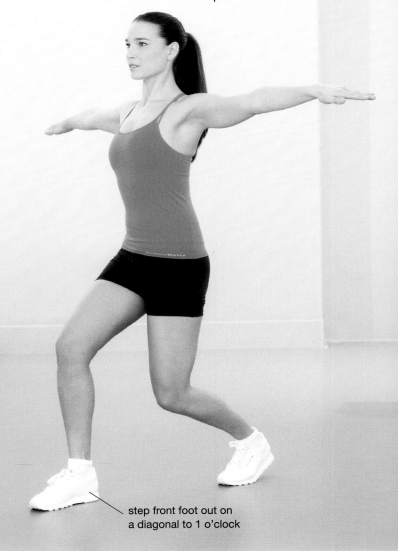

step front foot out on a diagonal to 1 o'clock

5a

Side lunge Stand with your feet parallel, hip width apart. Raise your arms to the sides at shoulder height, palms down. Keep your abdominals tight, hips square to the front, chest lifted. Draw your shoulder blades down and together as you prepare to lunge.

5b

Inhale and step your left leg out to the side (9 o'clock), bending your knee. At the same time reach your arms high, turning the palms in, and flex your torso towards the centre, bending sideways at the waist. Exhale and spring back to centre, rotating the palms down as you lower your arms to shoulder height. Alternate sides (lunge to 3 o'clock) for 8 reps (1 rep = both sides).

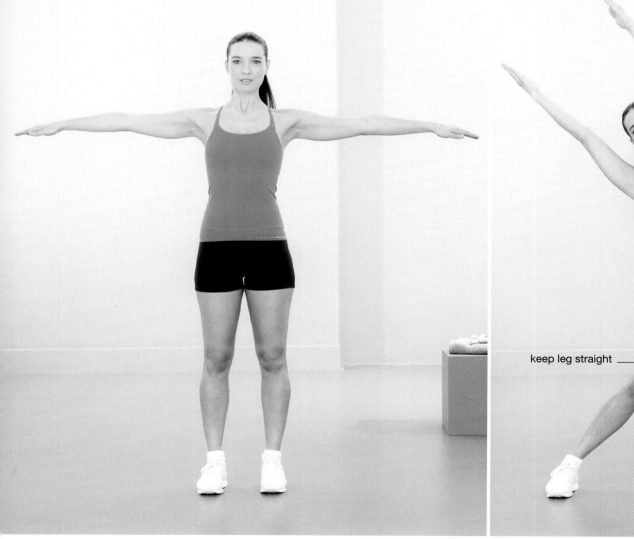

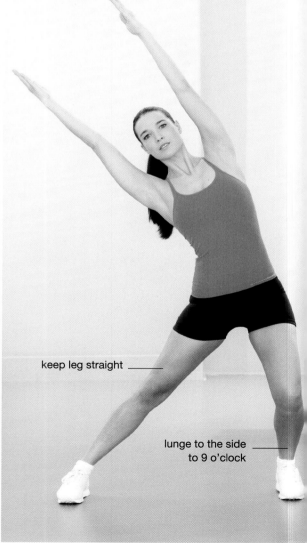

keep leg straight

lunge to the side to 9 o'clock

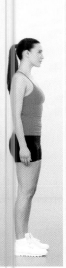

6 **Reverse lunge** Start in the center position, feet parallel, arms by your sides. Inhale as you lunge to the back (6 o'clock), landing on the ball of your foot, and bending both knees. At the same time, reach both arms high in front, palms in. Exhale and return to centre, arms by your sides. Repeat for 8 reps (1 rep = both sides). **Repeat Steps 5–1 (in reverse order) to complete your warm up.**

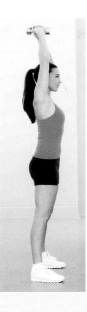

7 **Wood-chop squat** Pick up one large weight. Standing with your feet parallel, shoulder width apart, hold the weight overhead. Inhale as you squat, lowering the weight to your knees as if you are chopping wood. Exhale as you return to the starting position and repeat for 12 reps.

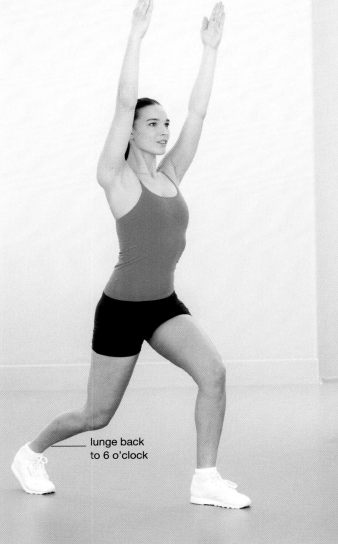

lunge back to 6 o'clock

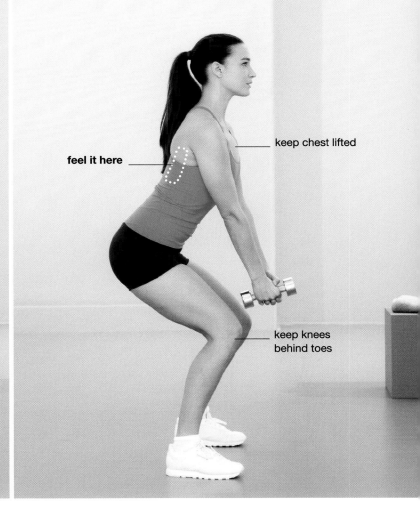

feel it here

keep chest lifted

keep knees behind toes

8a

Curtsy lunge Put down the weight for your first cardio interval. Stand with your feet parallel, hip width apart, knees soft. Raise your arms out to the sides at shoulder height, palms down. Keep your elbows slightly rounded. Stand tall, lengthening through your spine by lifting the top of your head towards the ceiling and engaging the abdominals.

8b

Step back on a diagonal, landing on the ball of your foot, heel lifted. Bend both knees and squeeze your shoulder blades together every time you curtsy. Keep your arms at shoulder height. Breathe naturally throughout. Repeat for 8 reps, alternating legs (1 rep = both sides).

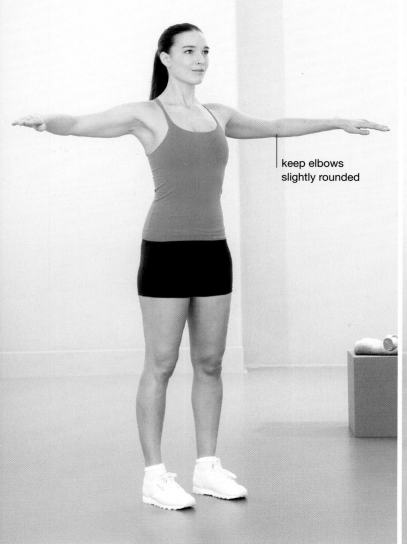

keep elbows
slightly rounded

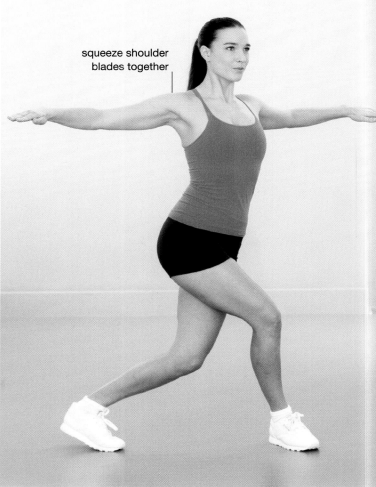

squeeze shoulder
blades together

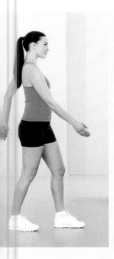

9a **Charleston lunge** Step forwards with the lead leg and kick the other leg in front of you, knee to hip height. Then swing the leg back and step in place. Swing your arms in opposition to your legs. Continue the movement with the Reverse lunge (see 9b).

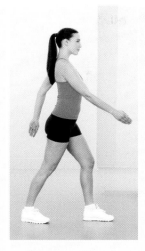

9b Reverse lunge with the lead leg. Continue a series of step, kick front (see 9a), step, lunge back. Swap arms with every leg change. Repeat 6 times. Change legs by substituting the last lunge with a step in place. Repeat the sequence 6 times on the other side.

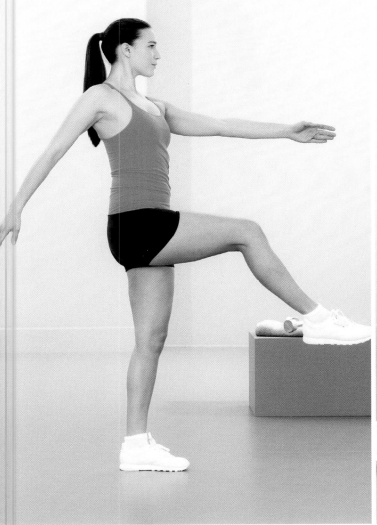

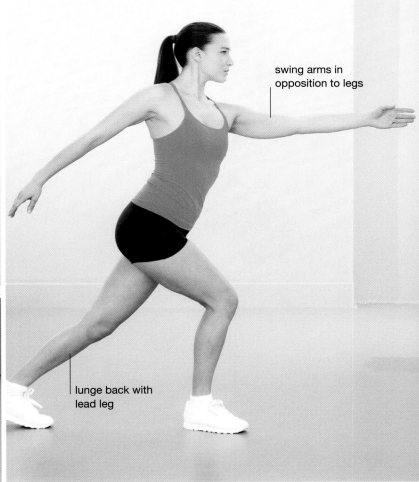

swing arms in opposition to legs

lunge back with lead leg

10a

Push-off lunge
Start from a staggered lunge position, your front knee over the ankle. Your back heel should lift easily. Reach your arms overhead on a diagonal, palms in. Centre your weight between your legs, torso square to the front, eyes looking forwards. Prepare to push off with your back foot.

10b

Push off with your back foot, shifting your weight to your front leg, and pump your knee to hip height. At the same time, bend your arms, pulling your elbows to your sides, hands to hip level. Balance for a moment on the supporting leg before lunging again. Repeat a total of 8 times, then change to the other side. Breathe naturally throughout. **You have now completed the cardio interval, which you will repeat after each resistance exercise.**

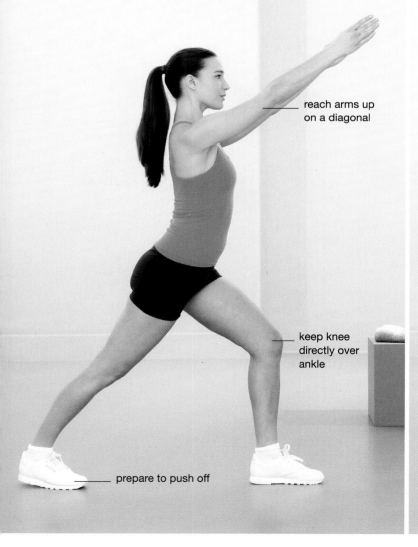

reach arms up
on a diagonal

keep knee
directly over
ankle

prepare to push off

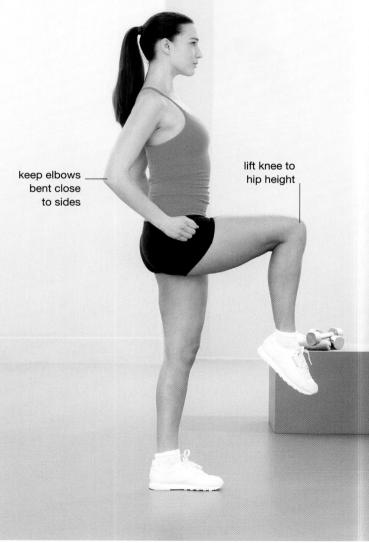

keep elbows
bent close
to sides

lift knee to
hip height

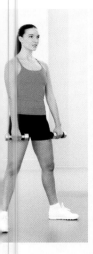

11 **Plié & row** Pick up two small weights. Stand with your legs turned out, slightly wider than shoulder width apart. Hold a weight in each hand, arms straight down, palms facing back. Inhale as you bend your knees over your toes and pull the weights to your chest, elbows bending out to the sides. Exhale and straighten up, lowering the weights. Move up and down 12 times. **Do your next cardio interval, Steps 8–10.**

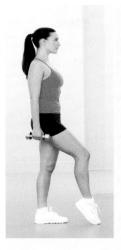

12 **Balance squat** Stand with all your weight on one leg, the other leg resting lightly to the front. Inhale, reach back with your hips and squat on the working leg. Exhale up. Repeat 12 times, then change sides. **Do your next cardio interval, Steps 8–10.**

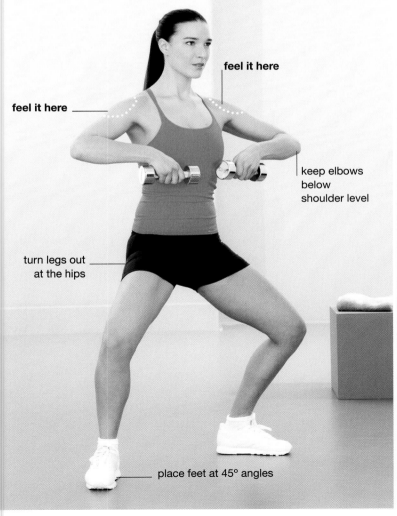

feel it here

feel it here

keep elbows below shoulder level

turn legs out at the hips

place feet at 45° angles

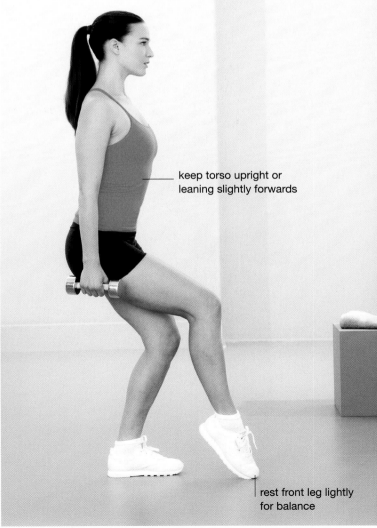

keep torso upright or leaning slightly forwards

rest front leg lightly for balance

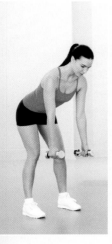

13a

Bent-over row
Pick up two weights. Stand with your feet parallel, shoulder width apart, holding a weight in each hand, arms by your sides, palms in. Bend your knees and hinge forwards from the hips, keeping your spine in neutral alignment. Draw your shoulder blades together and exhale as you lift the weights, bending your elbows until the upper arms are parallel to the floor.

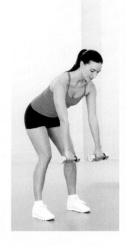

13b

Lower the weights to the starting position and rotate your arms so that your palms face back. Pull your shoulder blades together and exhale as you bend your elbows out to the sides until your upper arms are parallel to the floor. Do 8 reps, alternating the position of the arms. **Do your next cardio interval, Steps 8–10.**

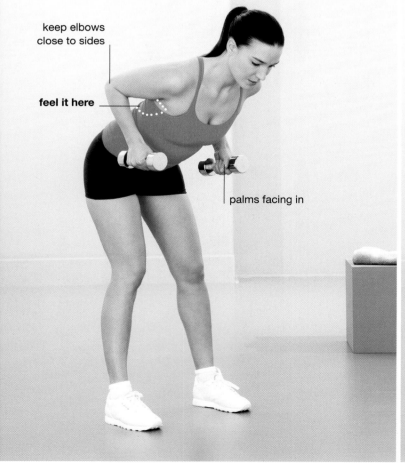

keep elbows close to sides

feel it here

palms facing in

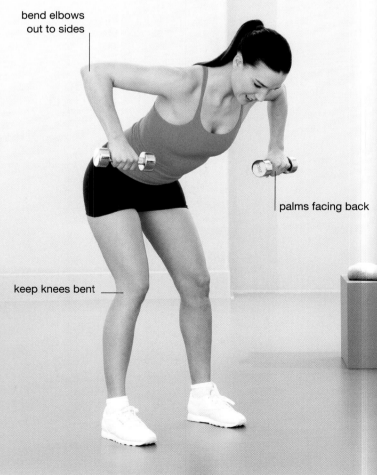

bend elbows out to sides

palms facing back

keep knees bent

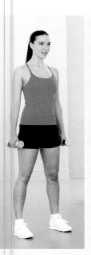

14a Lift & squat
Pick up two small weights. Stand feet parallel, shoulder width apart. Hold a weight in each hand, arms by your sides. Shift your weight to the balls of your feet and lift the heels high; at the same time, bend your elbows, lifting the weights towards your shoulders. Balance, then return to the starting position.

14b
Plant your heels on the floor, shift your weight back, and bend your knees into a squat. At the same time, raise your arms behind you, elbows straight. Straighten up, then repeat the combination of rising onto the balls of the feet followed by squatting for 8 reps. Breathe naturally throughout. **Do your next cardio interval, Steps 8–10.**

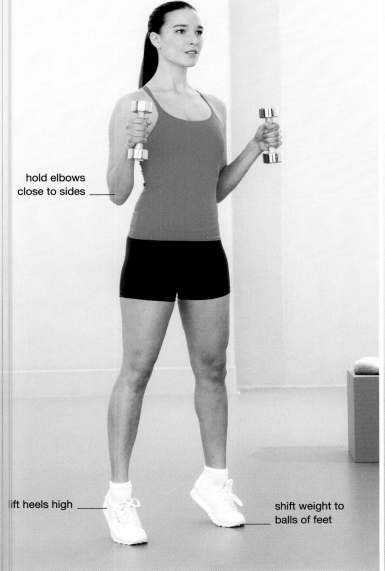

hold elbows close to sides

lift heels high

shift weight to balls of feet

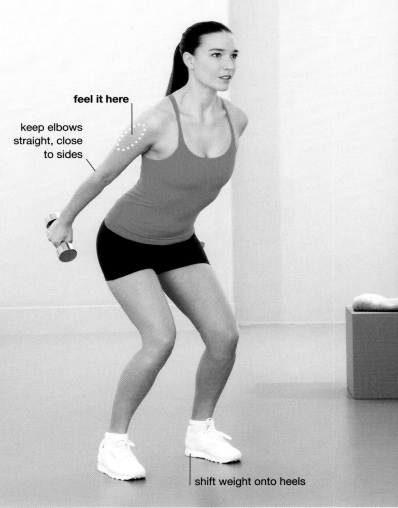

feel it here

keep elbows straight, close to sides

shift weight onto heels

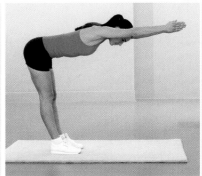

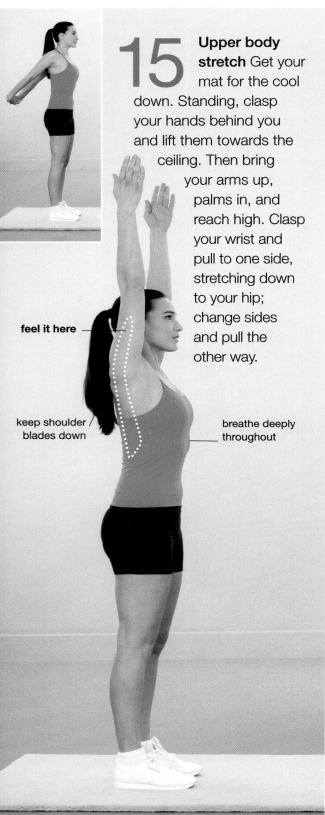

15 **Upper body stretch** Get your mat for the cool down. Standing, clasp your hands behind you and lift them towards the ceiling. Then bring your arms up, palms in, and reach high. Clasp your wrist and pull to one side, stretching down to your hip; change sides and pull the other way.

feel it here

keep shoulder blades down

breathe deeply throughout

16 **Upper body stretch/Down dog** Return to centre and hinge forwards from the hips; knees and back straight. Reach back with the hips, extending your arms forwards, lengthening the spine. Hold the stretch and breathe. Bend down, place your palms on the mat, and walk your hands into Down dog, reaching your hips upwards and pressing your heels towards the mat. If necessary, bend your knees to release hips and heels. Keep the breath flowing.

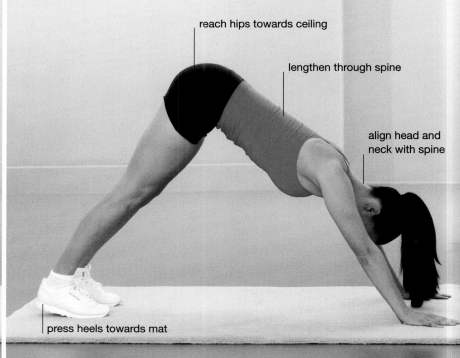

reach hips towards ceiling

lengthen through spine

align head and neck with spine

press heels towards mat

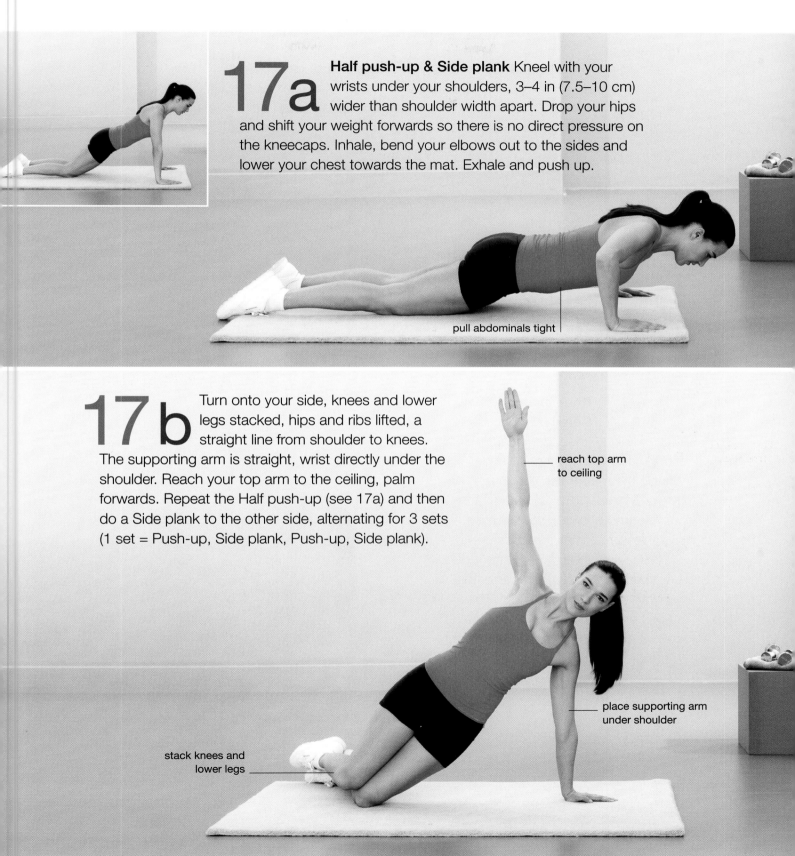

17a

Half push-up & Side plank Kneel with your wrists under your shoulders, 3–4 in (7.5–10 cm) wider than shoulder width apart. Drop your hips and shift your weight forwards so there is no direct pressure on the kneecaps. Inhale, bend your elbows out to the sides and lower your chest towards the mat. Exhale and push up.

pull abdominals tight

17b

Turn onto your side, knees and lower legs stacked, hips and ribs lifted, a straight line from shoulder to knees. The supporting arm is straight, wrist directly under the shoulder. Reach your top arm to the ceiling, palm forwards. Repeat the Half push-up (see 17a) and then do a Side plank to the other side, alternating for 3 sets (1 set = Push-up, Side plank, Push-up, Side plank).

reach top arm to ceiling

place supporting arm under shoulder

stack knees and lower legs

18 **Child's pose** Come onto your knees and sit back, reaching your hips towards your heels. At the same time, round forwards and reach your arms to the front, forehead to mat. Allow your body to relax and sink into the position.

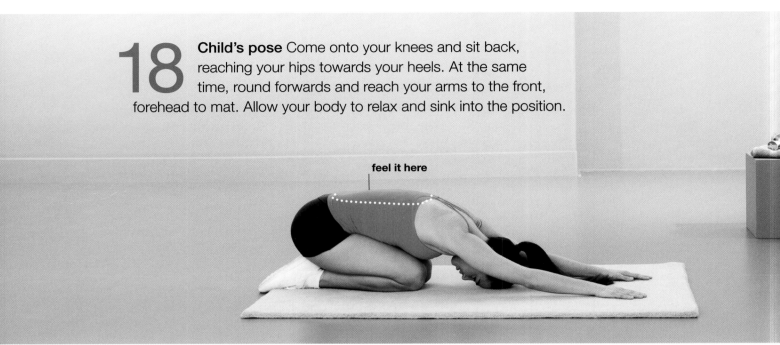

feel it here

19 **Kneeling lunge** Come up onto one knee, bending the other one in front of you, foot on the mat. Raise your arms overhead, palms in, head centred between your elbows. Press your hips forwards until you feel a stretch in the front of your hip, the hip flexor. Breathe into the stretch and hold. Then sit back into Child's pose (see above). Repeat the lunge on the other side.

keep hips square to front

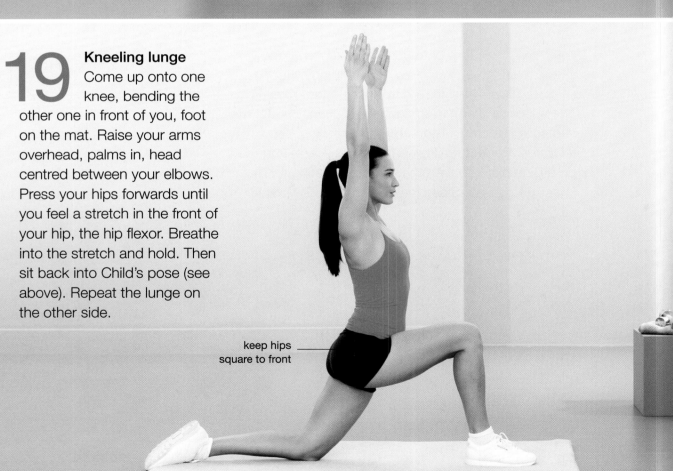

20a **Cross-legged stretch**
Sit back on your buttocks and cross your legs comfortably in front. Bend forwards from the hips with your back straight, keep the sitting bones anchored on the floor, and extend your arms to the front. Breathe deeply and relax into the position.

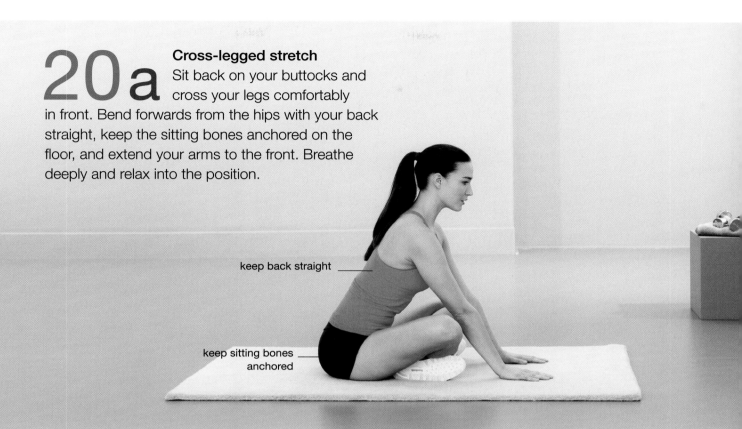

keep back straight _____

keep sitting bones _____
anchored

20b
Walk your hands to one side, turning your torso to face that knee. Hold the position briefly and breathe deeply, trying to relax more deeply into the position with each exhalation. Pass through centre and repeat on the other side. Remember to keep your sitting bones anchored throughout.

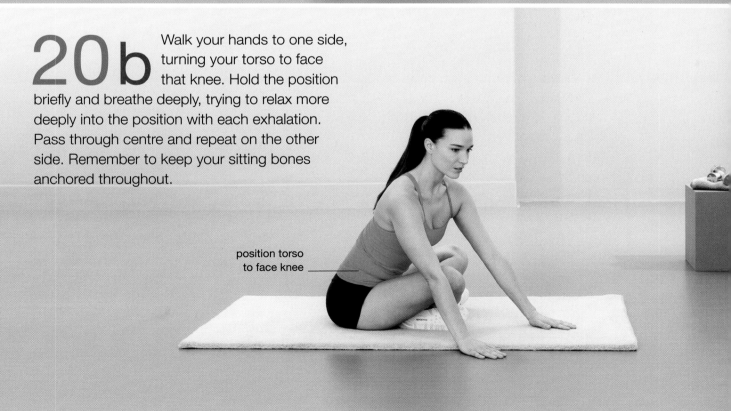

position torso
to face knee _____

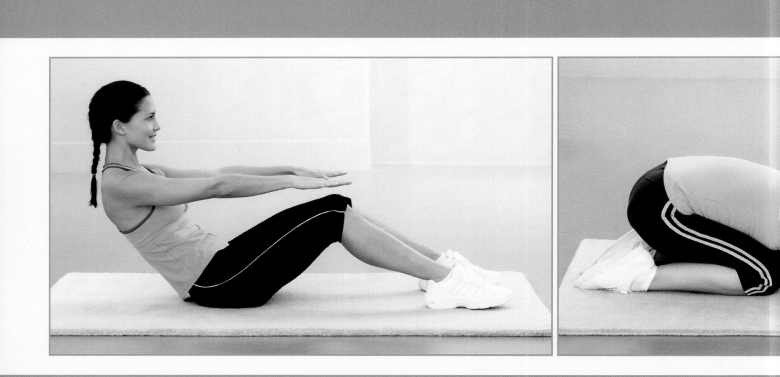

focus on

tum

Pick 8–10 exercises to work
the abdominal muscles for a
flatter belly and a trimmer waist

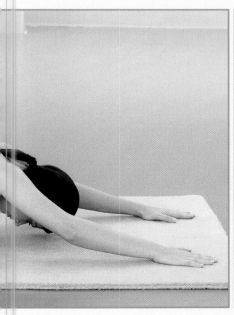
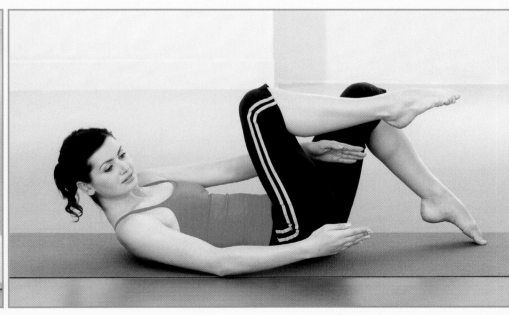

The crunch is the classic abs exercise, targeting the rectus abdominis muscle that runs from the sternum to the pubic bone. It is a versatile exercise, suitable for beginners or more advanced exercisers. It also ranks as one of the most effective for strengthening the abdomen.

The function of the rectus muscle is to flex the spine, and in the crunch you do not perform more than 30° of spinal flexion (which refers to how high you lift your upper torso off the floor), even if you can raise your torso higher. This range of motion isolates the muscle, keeping the work in the rectus. If you lift higher, as in a full sit-up, for example, you activate other muscles, primarily the hip flexors in the front of the thigh. In addition to being a more effective isolation exercise than the full sit-up, the crunch places less stress on the low back and is therefore safer.

It is useful to have an objective measure of your starting level of abdominal fitness. Together with your health and medical information, a fitness assessment helps define your goals in an exercise programme. Establishing a baseline also enables you to measure your improvement. One way to measure muscular fitness is to count how many repetitions you can perform. Do the crunch test as described below. Write down your results, make a note of the date, and after two months of training, repeat the assessment.

To get the most from your workout, use proper form and execution of the crunch. Concentrate on perfecting the technique and apply it to each repetition. Mental focus also enhances the outcome – think about feeling the abdominal muscle tightening, strength coming from the core centre, lifting from the chest, head relaxed in your hands.

Preparation for the crunch

Make a cradle for your head by spreading your fingertips and supporting the base of your skull. Bend your fingers slightly and let the weight of your head rest in your hands. Keep your chin lifted, as if you were holding an orange under it (measure the distance with your fist, as in the photograph on p79, top left). Keep your elbows wide to reduce any tendency to pull on your neck.

With your low back relaxed in neutral alignment (see p80), engage the rectus abdominis by tightening the connection between the ribs and the hips. Keep tension in the muscle as you lift your chest to the ceiling, shoulder blades clearing the floor. Maintain the tension as you lower your

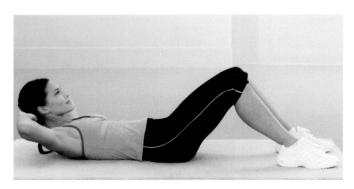

Neutral crunch
Count how many neutral crunches you can do consecutively without resting. Remember, this is not a full sit-up. Lift your shoulders no higher than 30° off the mat.

Your score

Excellent	50 or more
Good	35–49 reps
Fair	20–34 reps
Poor	fewer than 20 reps

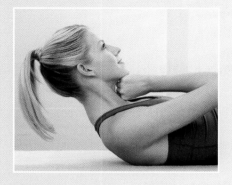

Fist under chin Use your fist under your chin to gauge the correct alignment of the head. Always think, 'Chin up'.

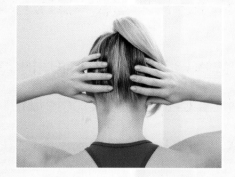

Position of hands on head Spread your fingers at the base of your skull to create a cradle for holding your head. Remember to relax your neck in your hands.

shoulder blades to the floor and, without resting at the bottom, immediately repeat the lift. Keep drawing the ribs to the pelvis – think of 'scooping' out the abdomen. Learn to breathe while you are drawing in, holding tension in the muscle – inhale first, then exhale as you lift up. Use slow, controlled movements and work the entire range of motion. It's quality not quantity that counts!

The weight of your head and upper torso provide resistance in the crunch.

You can increase the intensity by slowing the action, adding holds (as in the Long crunch, p83) and the Diamond crunch, p92), or by adding external resistance by placing a fitness ball between your knees when performing exercises such as the Reverse Crunch (p93). You can increase the resistance if you wish by using a weighted ball of 1.4–1.8kg (3–4 lbs) to help with muscle strengthening. My favourite weighted balls are filled with gel.

Connecting ribs to hips Set your abs before you move. Think of connecting the ribs to the hips. Maintain this connection, drawing ribs to pelvis, while you perform crunches.

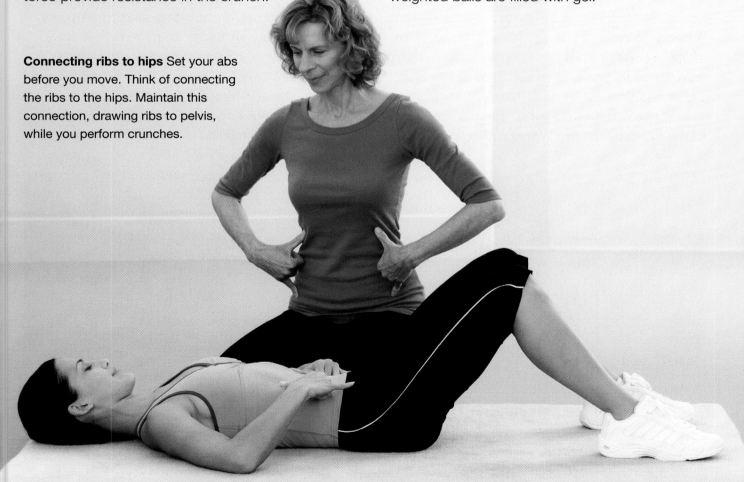

The deepest abdominal muscle, the transversus abdominis, is a flat, horizontal band of muscle that encircles the waist from front to back. Toning it creates a natural corset-like effect of narrowing the waist, flattening the abdomen and supporting the low back.

The transversus abdominis plays a significant role in core strength. It functions to stabilize the pelvis and maintain the small curve in the low back, which affects your posture and alignment in all positions against gravity, whether you are stationary or moving. In fitness training, sports activities and everyday life, a stable core provides stability for the trunk, which increases the control of the movement you are performing.

A few simple exercises can help you to develop body awareness of your deep abdominals. Belly breathing is key here because the transversus abdominis functions (together with the obliques) to compress the abdomen when you exhale. Practise a belly breath; inhale, fill the belly with air, then exhale forcefully by pulling the abdominals tight (think 'navel to spine'), then push the air out.

Next, find your own neutral spine alignment, the place where your spine rests while preserving all its natural curves. You should have a slight curve in the low back – with just enough space to slip your hand in if you are standing straight with your back against a wall. It may be more difficult to establish the neutral position when lying down, but it is halfway between a full arch and a flat-back position. The correct alignment of the low back, neither flattened nor arched, will allow you to recruit your core muscles most effectively.

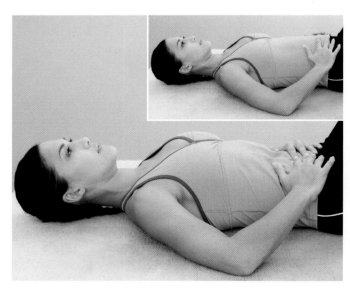

Belly breaths Place your hands on your belly to feel the action of the abdominals as they expand to take the air in (inset) and compress to push the air out.

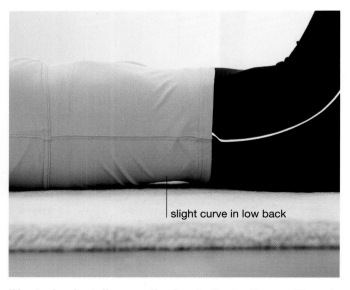

slight curve in low back

'Neutral spine alignment' refers to the resting position of the spine with all its natural curves in place. The low back retains its slight curve and is neither arched nor flattened.

▶▶▶ tips for **core training**

- **Warm up the pelvis** Do 10 Pelvic tilts (see below) with belly breaths to rehearse the breathing, practise abdominal compression and move the pelvis in a controlled way.

- **Active stabilization** Do a strong Pelvic tilt and release halfway, keeping the abdominals engaged, low back relaxed. With the pelvis stabilized like this, breathe naturally.

- **Monitor the position of the pelvis** Place your fingers under your sacrum to make sure it stays level.

The Pelvic tilt (see p82) can be used as a technique to learn how to actively stabilize the pelvis in neutral spine alignment. To perform a Pelvic tilt, combine a belly breath with a slight rotation of the pelvis – inhale, expand the belly as you take in the air; exhale, compress the abdomen and press the low back to the floor. Now, keep your abdominals tight and release the Pelvic tilt halfway. Relax the low back, allowing the slight natural curve. The abdominals should remain taut or stiff to the touch.

To assess the strength of the transversus abdominis, we challenge its ability to stabilize the pelvis against the changing resistance of various leg movements. There are three levels of difficulty, as shown on the right. All variations are performed lying on your back, with your arms resting to the sides, palms up, to minimize any assistance from the upper body. As you add the leg movements, use your abs to keep your low back from arching and your hips from rocking side to side. A good way to monitor how you are doing is to place your fingers under your pelvis and feel the two bumps on either side of your sacrum just below your waist. As you raise and lower your legs, make sure that the pelvis stays level, exerting even pressure on your fingers, and doesn't lift up on either side.

Assessing the strength of the **transversus abdominis**

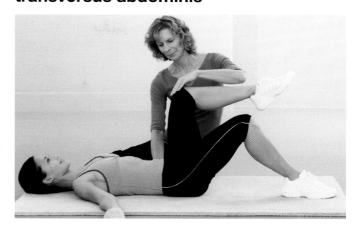

Beginner level Engage the abs, lift one leg at a time, keeping the right angle at the knee, then lower the leg back to the floor. Alternate sides for 10 reps.

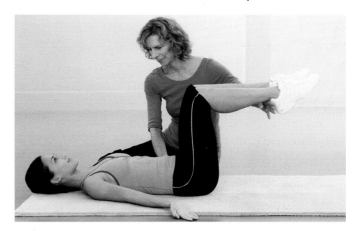

Intermediate level Come into 90–90, one leg at a time, right angles at hips and knees, low back in neutral alignment. Hold this position for 30 seconds or more.

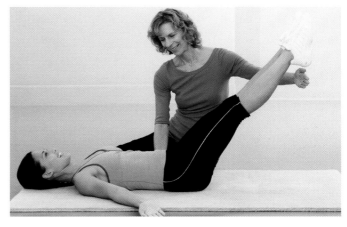

Advanced level From 90–90, straighten both legs to the ceiling and lower them towards the floor, as far as you can without arching the low back.

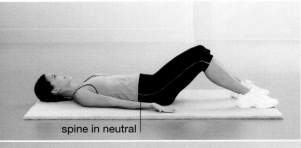

spine in neutral

Pelvic tilt

Stay on your back with bent knees and arms by your sides, palms up. Inhale and fill your belly with air. Now exhale forcefully, pulling your abs in tight and, with one fluid motion, flatten your low back to the floor. Hold for a moment, then release. Repeat 10 times.

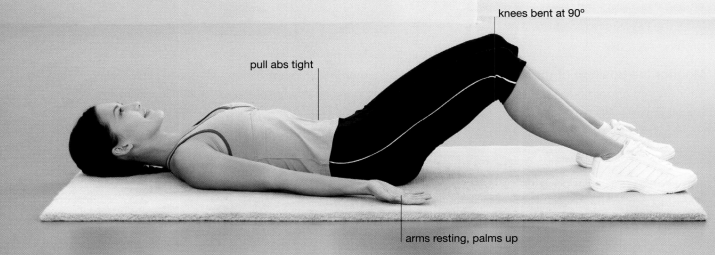

knees bent at 90°

pull abs tight

arms resting, palms up

Short crunch

Move your feet in close to your buttocks, connect the ribs to the hips, then place your hands behind your head. Inhale first, then exhale, scooping out your abs, navel to spine, as you lift your shoulder blades 30° off the floor. Release, slowly lowering your shoulders (but not your head) to the floor. Repeat 10 times.

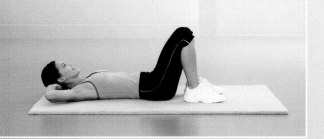

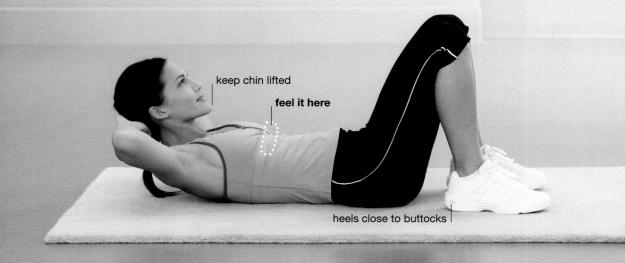

keep chin lifted

feel it here

heels close to buttocks

Neutral crunch

Move your feet forwards until your knees are bent at 90°. Tighten your abs and prepare to pick up the pace. Continue to lift and lower your shoulders rhythmically, exhaling as you lift and inhaling as you release, maintaining tension in your abs throughout the movement. Repeat 10 times.

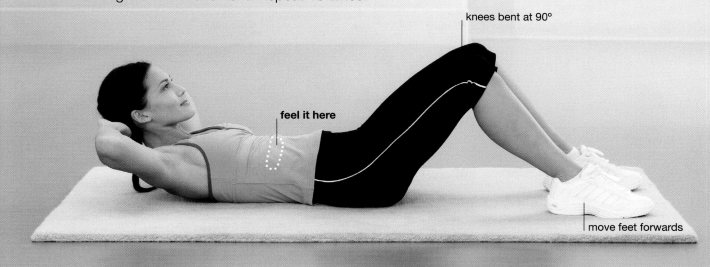

knees bent at 90°

feel it here

move feet forwards

Long crunch

Extend your legs, keeping a slight bend in your knees. Inhale first, then exhale and pull *in* as you crunch *up*. Release slowly. Learn to keep tension in the muscle while you continue to breathe. Repeat 10 times, then stretch out, arms and legs long.

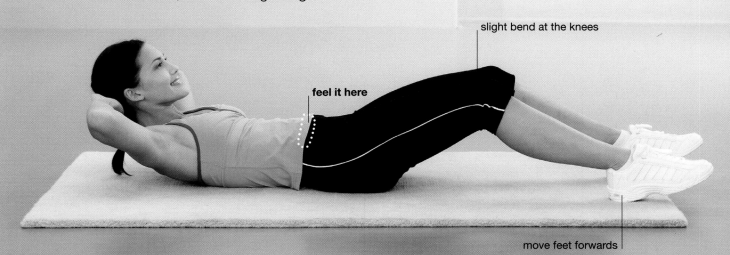

slight bend at the knees

feel it here

move feet forwards

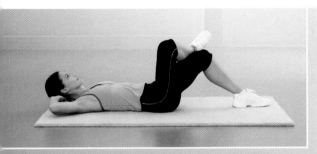

Side crunch

Move your feet in closer to create a 90° bend at the knees, then cross one ankle over the opposite knee, hands behind your head. With elbows wide, inhale, then exhale and twist one shoulder towards the opposite knee. Pause, then slowly release without resting your head on the floor. Repeat 5 times on each side.

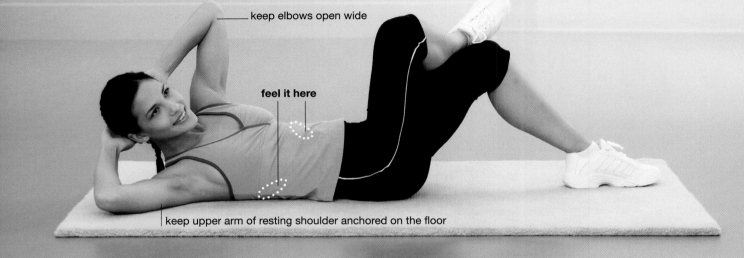

keep elbows open wide

feel it here

keep upper arm of resting shoulder anchored on the floor

Lengthening stretch

Reach out long, extending your arms and legs. Take a deep breath in and stretch out as far as you can. Cross one ankle over the other and take the wrist on the same side in your other hand. Pull to the opposite side, stretching out the entire side of your torso. Pause, then change sides and repeat.

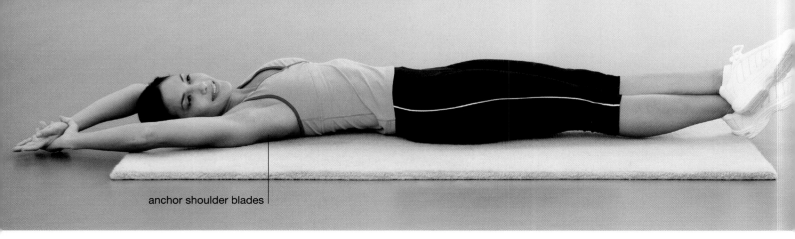

anchor shoulder blades

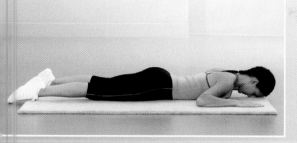

Press-up

Lie face down, arms bent in the shape of a 'W', forearms resting on the floor, palms down. Squeeze your shoulder blades down and together. Lengthen through your torso, reaching the top of your head forwards. Exhale as you lift your head and shoulders off the floor without using any strength from your arms. Keep your nose down. Repeat 8 times.

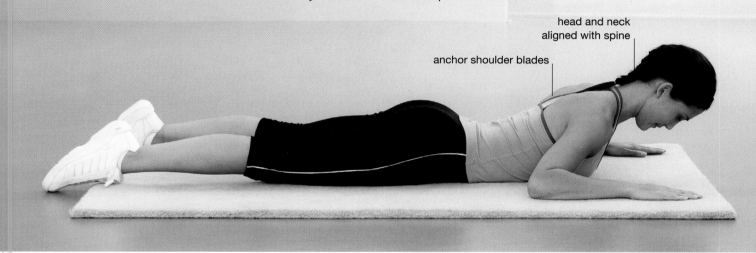

head and neck
aligned with spine

anchor shoulder blades

Sphinx

Lie face down, elbows bent with forearms resting on the floor. Anchor your shoulder blades as you lift your chest, sliding your elbows forwards to be directly under your shoulders. Pull your ribs away from your hips, stretching your abdomen. With your shoulders square to the front, turn your head to one side and hold; then to the other.

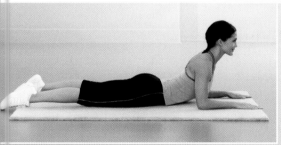

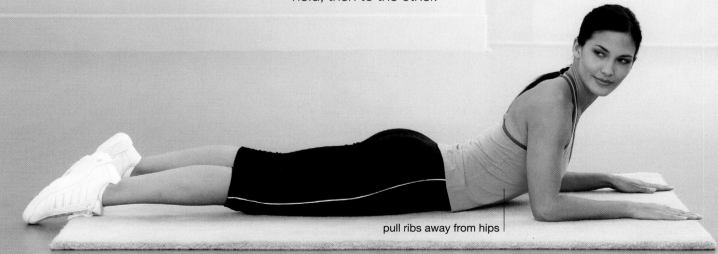

pull ribs away from hips

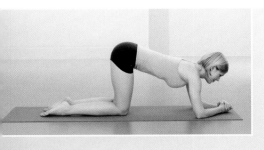

Forearm plank

a Go onto the forearms and knees. Clasp your hands in front of you. Lift your abs and tighten your glutes as you step one leg back at a time to create a forearm plank.

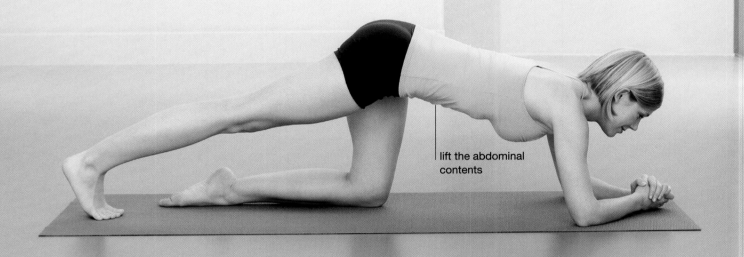

lift the abdominal contents

b Pull up the abs and press the pubic bone down towards the floor. Curl the tailbone under to firmly lock the hips. Take 2 breaths. Bend the knees back to kneeling, then repeat the exercise. Relax.

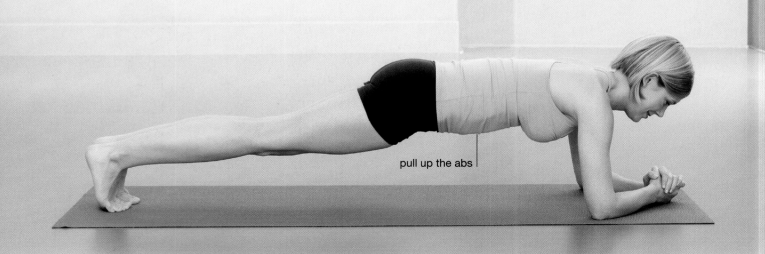

pull up the abs

Advancing frogs

a Come onto your hands and knees, open your knees, reach your arms forwards, and squat back, bringing your hips close to your heels. Support your back by lifting the abs. Stay for 2 breath cycles.

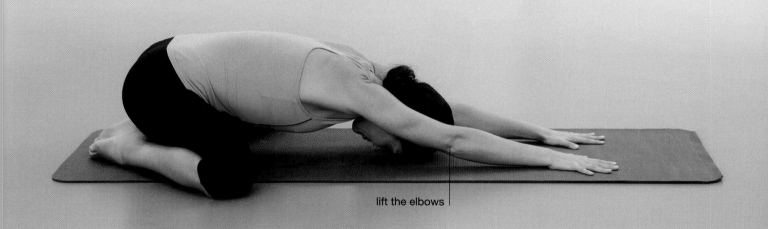

lift the elbows

b Move your torso and arms forwards, and come up on your forearms. Actively press the inner edges of your heels into the floor. Your heels will come apart. Scoop in your abs to avoid slumping in the low back. Stay for 2 breath cycles.

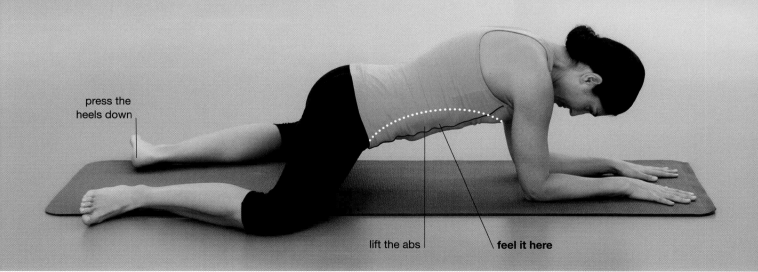

press the heels down

lift the abs

feel it here

Puppy dog abs

a Lie on your back with your knees bent and arms by your sides. Hold your abs firm and lift your legs up so your shins are parallel to the floor. Bend your elbows, take your upper arms off the floor and face your palms upwards. This 'puppy dog' position makes your core muscles work.

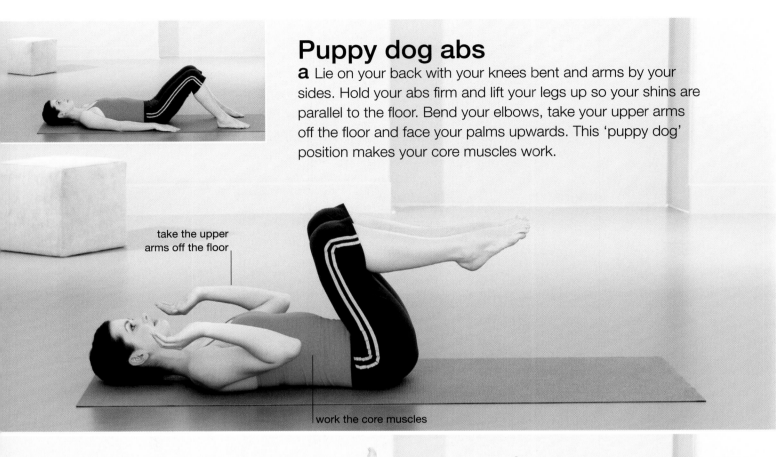

take the upper arms off the floor

work the core muscles

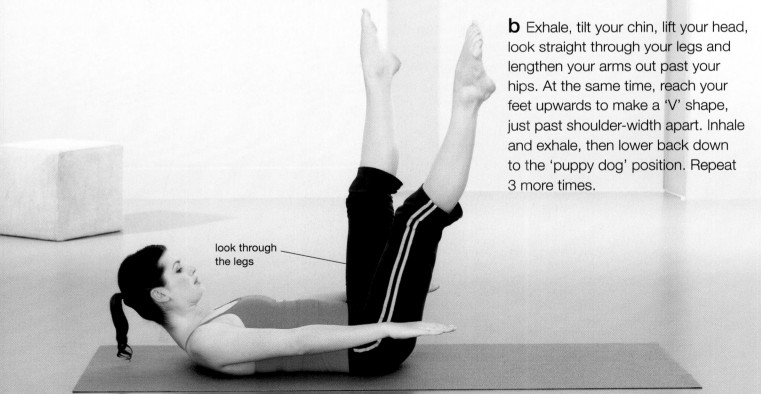

b Exhale, tilt your chin, lift your head, look straight through your legs and lengthen your arms out past your hips. At the same time, reach your feet upwards to make a 'V' shape, just past shoulder-width apart. Inhale and exhale, then lower back down to the 'puppy dog' position. Repeat 3 more times.

look through the legs

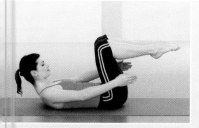

Toe touches

a Lie down with your knees bent. Exhale, curl up your upper body, reach your hands out past your thighs and take your feet off the floor. Look along your body. Take your left arm between your legs, reaching ahead with your middle fingers. Now lightly touch the toes of your left foot to the floor.

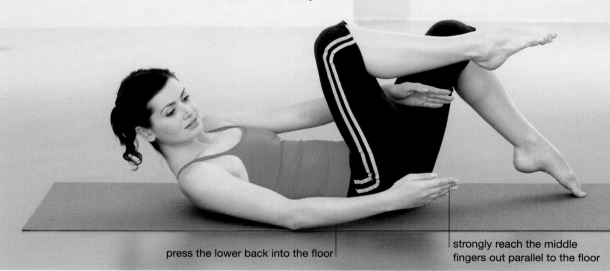

press the lower back into the floor

strongly reach the middle fingers out parallel to the floor

b Simultaneously touch the right foot to the floor as you raise the left. Alternate toe touches for 16 reps. Place the right arm between the legs and alternate toe touches for 16 more reps. To end, hold both legs and arms up and increase the pull of the middle fingers.

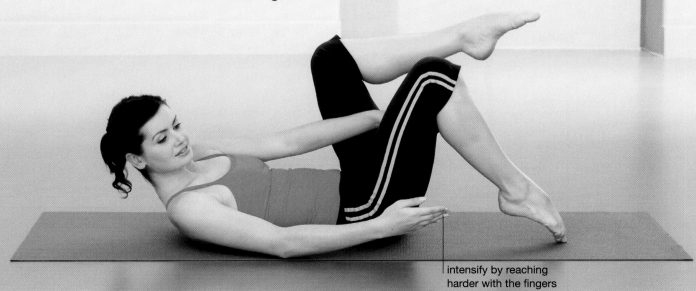

intensify by reaching harder with the fingers

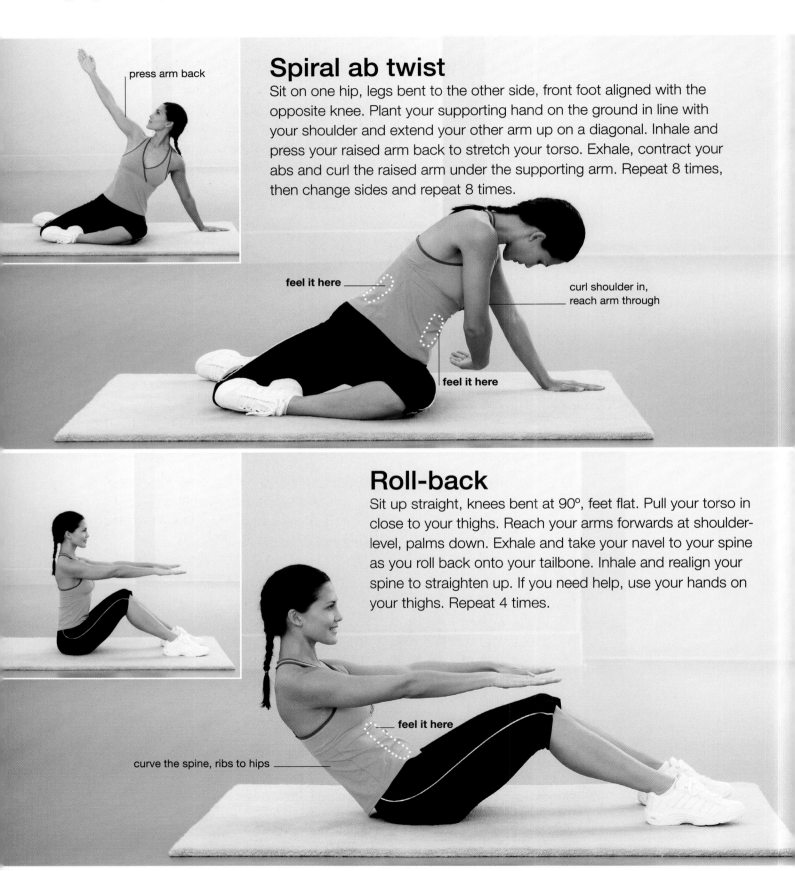

press arm back

Spiral ab twist

Sit on one hip, legs bent to the other side, front foot aligned with the opposite knee. Plant your supporting hand on the ground in line with your shoulder and extend your other arm up on a diagonal. Inhale and press your raised arm back to stretch your torso. Exhale, contract your abs and curl the raised arm under the supporting arm. Repeat 8 times, then change sides and repeat 8 times.

feel it here

curl shoulder in, reach arm through

feel it here

Roll-back

Sit up straight, knees bent at 90°, feet flat. Pull your torso in close to your thighs. Reach your arms forwards at shoulder-level, palms down. Exhale and take your navel to your spine as you roll back onto your tailbone. Inhale and realign your spine to straighten up. If you need help, use your hands on your thighs. Repeat 4 times.

feel it here

curve the spine, ribs to hips

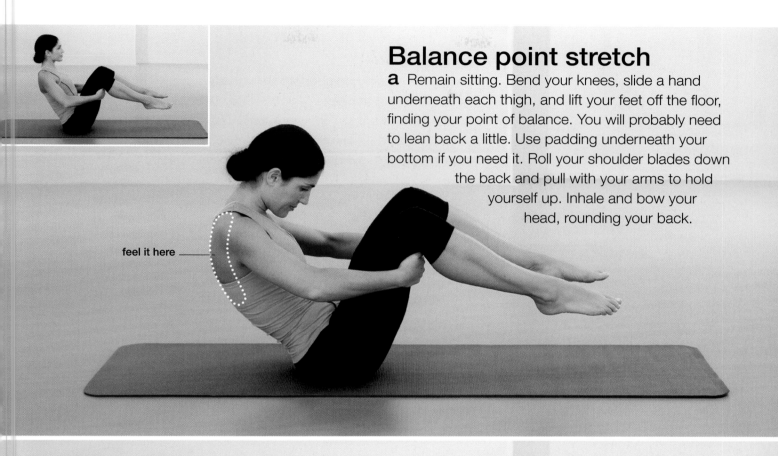

Balance point stretch

a Remain sitting. Bend your knees, slide a hand underneath each thigh, and lift your feet off the floor, finding your point of balance. You will probably need to lean back a little. Use padding underneath your bottom if you need it. Roll your shoulder blades down the back and pull with your arms to hold yourself up. Inhale and bow your head, rounding your back.

feel it here

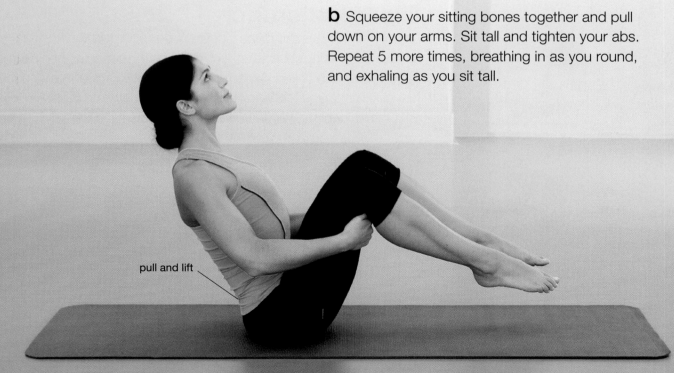

b Squeeze your sitting bones together and pull down on your arms. Sit tall and tighten your abs. Repeat 5 more times, breathing in as you round, and exhaling as you sit tall.

pull and lift

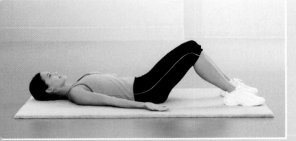

Bridge

Feet on the floor, knees bent at 90°, do a strong Pelvic tilt (see p82). Then, starting at the base of your spine, peel your back off the floor, one vertebra at a time, until your torso forms a straight line from knees to shoulders. Inhale as you release down, rolling through the curve in your low back. Repeat 5 times.

torso aligned from shoulders to knees

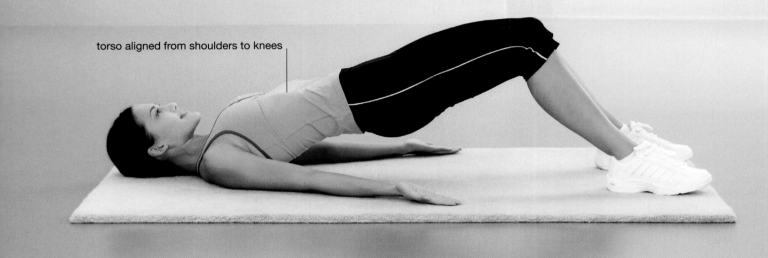

Diamond crunch

Lie with your knees out to the sides, soles of your feet together, as close to your body as possible. Connect your ribs to your hips, then rest your head in your hands and tighten your abs. Exhale as you lift your shoulder blades. Extend your arms towards your feet, crunching up higher. Return your hands behind your head, then lower to the floor. Repeat 6 times.

crunch higher as you reach

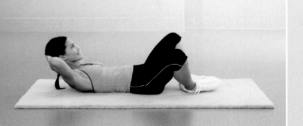

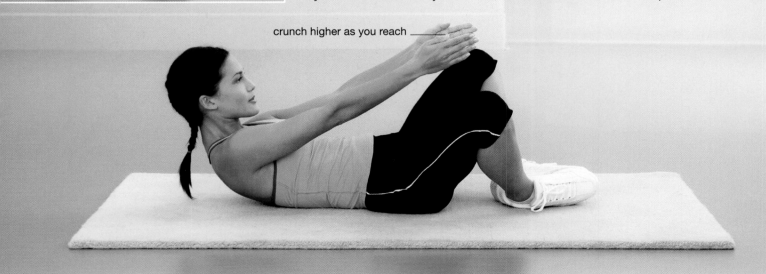

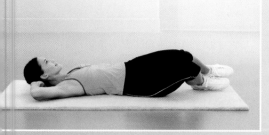

Torso twist

Feet on the floor, knees bent at 90°, place your hands behind head. Bring your legs together, knees and feet touching. Tighten your abs and slowly rotate your pelvis to one side, moving your knees halfway to the floor. Inhale, then exhale and crunch up towards the ceiling 10 times. Relax your knees to the floor and stretch for a moment, then repeat to the other side.

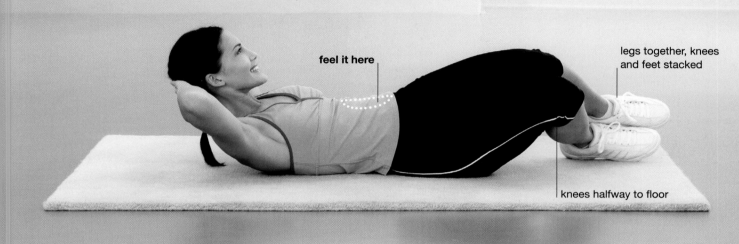

feel it here

legs together, knees and feet stacked

knees halfway to floor

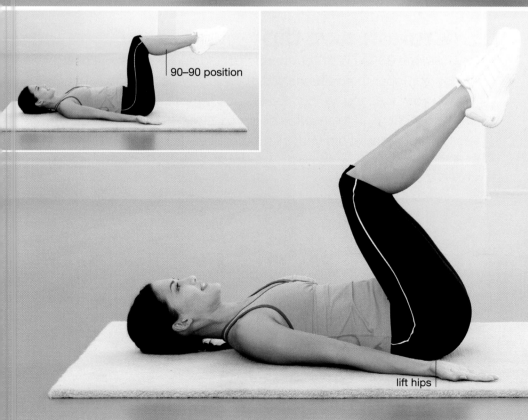

90–90 position

lift hips

Reverse crunch

Come into 90–90 with your legs raised with right angles at hips and knees, and arms resting by your sides, palms up. Inhale, then exhale and pull your navel towards your spine, drawing your pelvis towards your rib cage and lifting your hips. Use control to avoid swinging your legs with momentum. Repeat a total of 10 times.

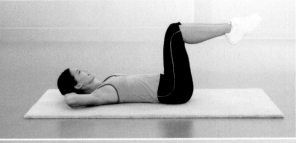

90–90 crunch

Still in 90–90, place your hands behind your head and tighten the connection between your ribs and your hips. Exhale as you lift your shoulder blades, eyes on the ceiling, chin lifted. Repeat 10 times. When you have finished, hug your knees into your chest and rest.

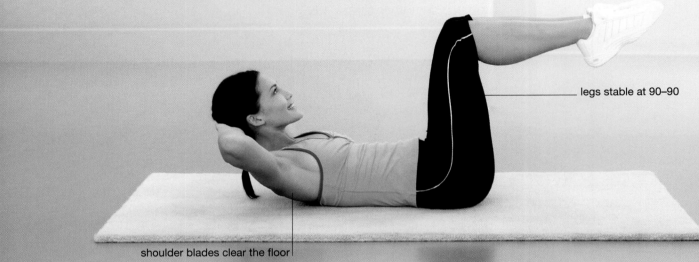

legs stable at 90–90

shoulder blades clear the floor

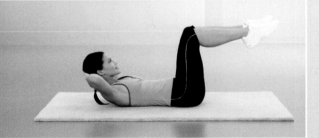

Crunch and dip

Resume 90–90 with your hands behind your head, exhale and do an upper torso crunch (inset). Hold it while you inhale and dip your toes to the floor. Exhale and return legs to 90–90, then inhale and release the crunch. Repeat 10 times, then hug your knees into your chest for a breather.

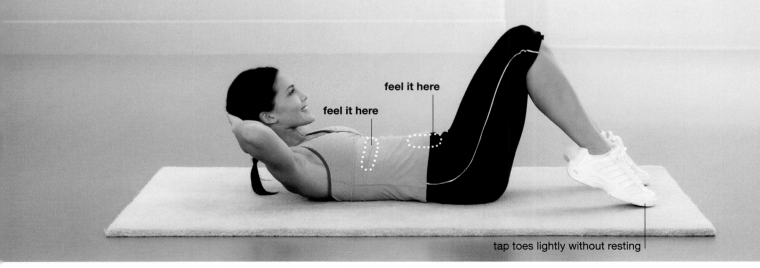

feel it here

feel it here

tap toes lightly without resting

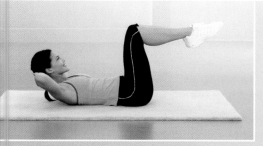

Bicycle

Return to 90–90, hands behind your head. Start with an upper torso crunch (inset), then exhale as you twist one elbow to the opposite knee, bringing your knee into your chest and extending your other leg towards the floor. Inhale back to centre and go to the other side. Alternate sides for 5 reps, keeping your shoulder blades lifted. Reach out long to stretch.

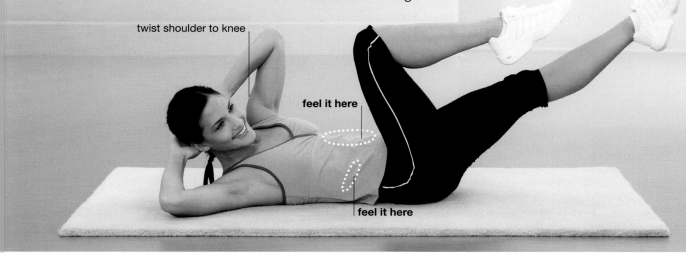

twist shoulder to knee

feel it here

feel it here

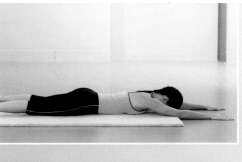

Arm and leg lift

Lying face down, extend your arms, palms down. Scoop in your abs and press your pubic bone into the floor. With your forehead still resting, exhale and lift one arm and the opposite leg, lengthening the limbs as you lift up. Repeat for 5 reps.

lengthen as you lift

feel it here

fully extend arm

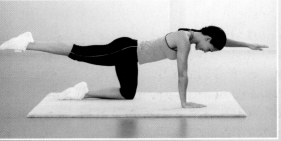

Kneeling lift

Kneel on all fours, wrists under shoulders, knees under hips. Extend one leg to hip-height, then lift the opposite arm to shoulder level. Stabilize the supporting arm by spreading your fingers and pushing into your thumb and index finger. Hold, then lower and lift your limbs 6 times, then hold again. Repeat on the other side.

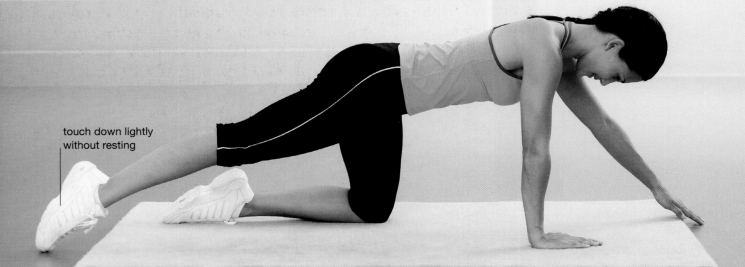

touch down lightly without resting

Forearm plank plus

From a forearm plank (see p10), lower both knees simultaneously 4 times. Then lower one knee at a time, alternating sides for 4 reps. If you are fatiguing, just try to hold the forearm plank. Breathe naturally throughout.

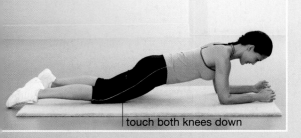

touch both knees down

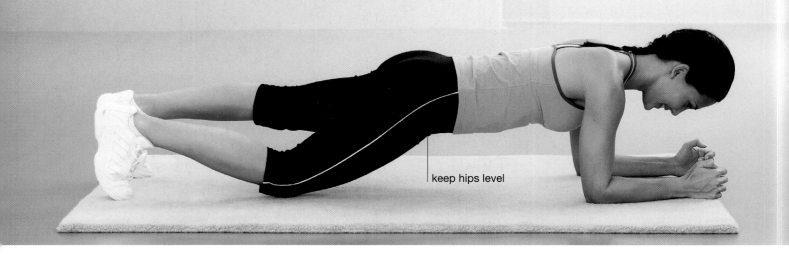

keep hips level

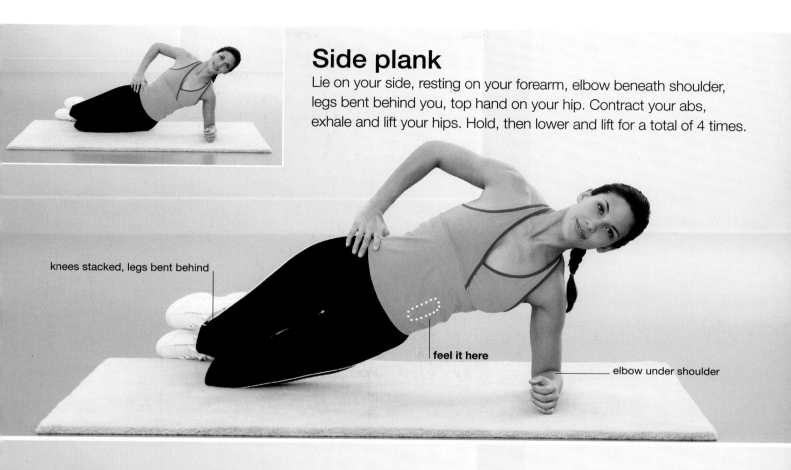

Side plank

Lie on your side, resting on your forearm, elbow beneath shoulder, legs bent behind you, top hand on your hip. Contract your abs, exhale and lift your hips. Hold, then lower and lift for a total of 4 times.

knees stacked, legs bent behind

feel it here

elbow under shoulder

Side plank with clam

Now add a challenging 'clam'. Open and close your top knee 4 times, keeping your rib cage lifted and the shoulder of your supporting arm down. Breathe naturally. Repeat Side plank and Side plank with clam on the other side.

keep hips stable

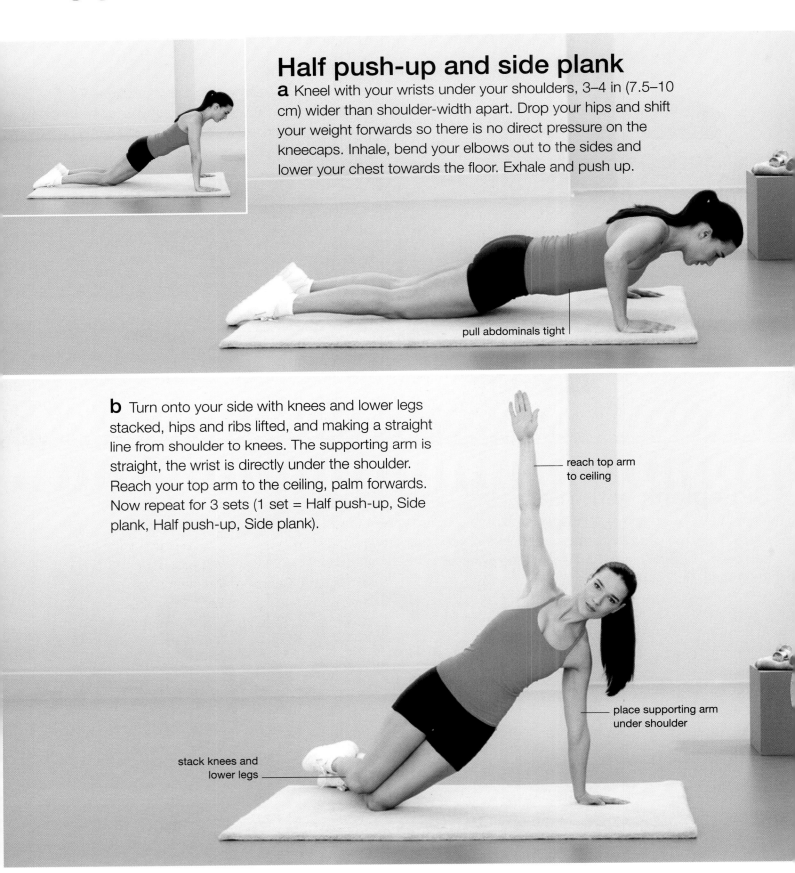

Half push-up and side plank

a Kneel with your wrists under your shoulders, 3–4 in (7.5–10 cm) wider than shoulder-width apart. Drop your hips and shift your weight forwards so there is no direct pressure on the kneecaps. Inhale, bend your elbows out to the sides and lower your chest towards the floor. Exhale and push up.

pull abdominals tight

b Turn onto your side with knees and lower legs stacked, hips and ribs lifted, and making a straight line from shoulder to knees. The supporting arm is straight, the wrist is directly under the shoulder. Reach your top arm to the ceiling, palm forwards. Now repeat for 3 sets (1 set = Half push-up, Side plank, Half push-up, Side plank).

reach top arm to ceiling

place supporting arm under shoulder

stack knees and lower legs

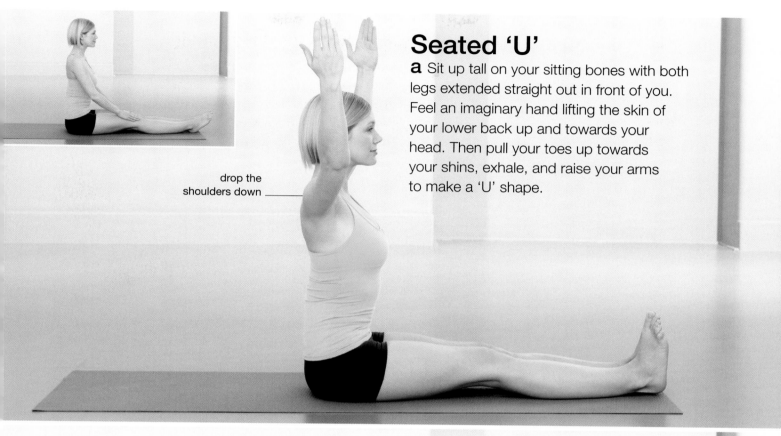

drop the
shoulders down

Seated 'U'

a Sit up tall on your sitting bones with both legs extended straight out in front of you. Feel an imaginary hand lifting the skin of your lower back up and towards your head. Then pull your toes up towards your shins, exhale, and raise your arms to make a 'U' shape.

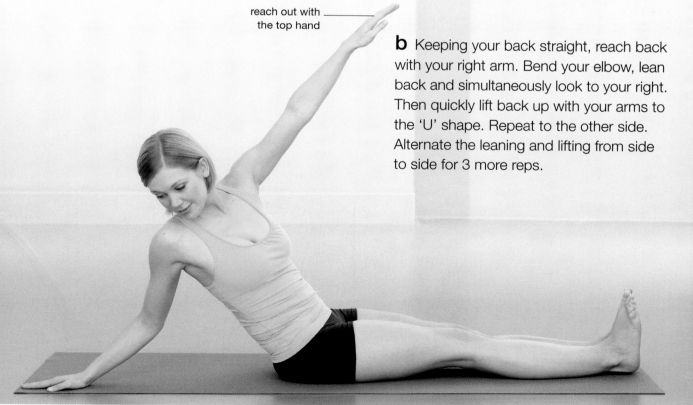

reach out with
the top hand

b Keeping your back straight, reach back with your right arm. Bend your elbow, lean back and simultaneously look to your right. Then quickly lift back up with your arms to the 'U' shape. Repeat to the other side. Alternate the leaning and lifting from side to side for 3 more reps.

Spinal twist

Lie on your back, with both knees bent and your feet on the floor to start your cool-down. Stretch your arms out in line with your shoulders, palms down. Drop your knees to one side and turn your head in the opposite direction. Breathe deeply.

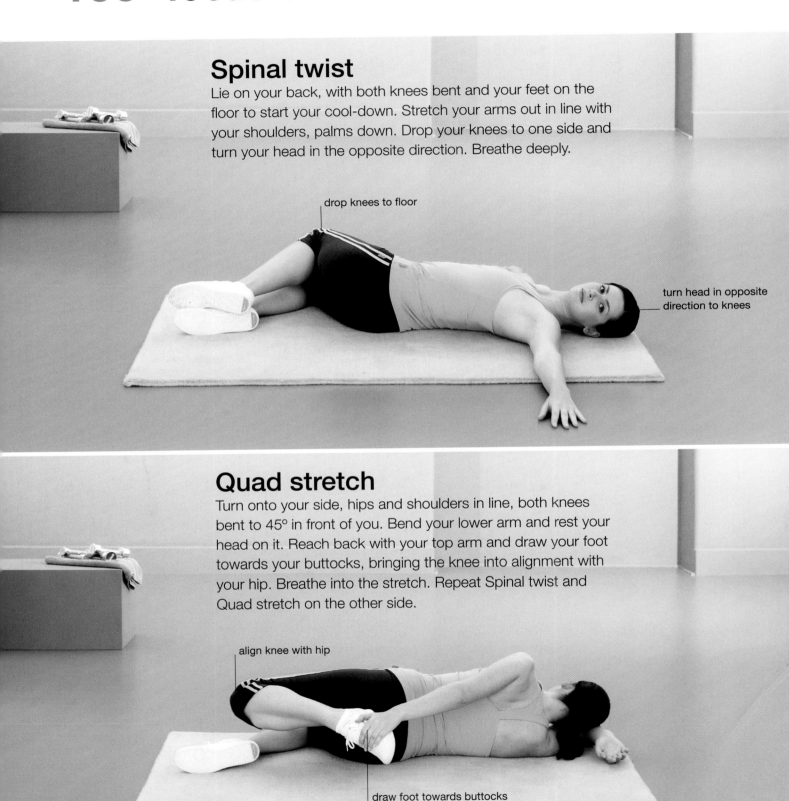

drop knees to floor

turn head in opposite direction to knees

Quad stretch

Turn onto your side, hips and shoulders in line, both knees bent to 45° in front of you. Bend your lower arm and rest your head on it. Reach back with your top arm and draw your foot towards your buttocks, bringing the knee into alignment with your hip. Breathe into the stretch. Repeat Spinal twist and Quad stretch on the other side.

align knee with hip

draw foot towards buttocks

Sphinx

Roll onto your front. Bend your elbows and rest your forearms on the mat. Draw your shoulder blades down as you lift your chest, sliding your elbows forwards to be directly under your shoulders. Turn your head to one side, then the other, to stretch the neck. Hold each position for a couple of breaths, breathing naturally throughout.

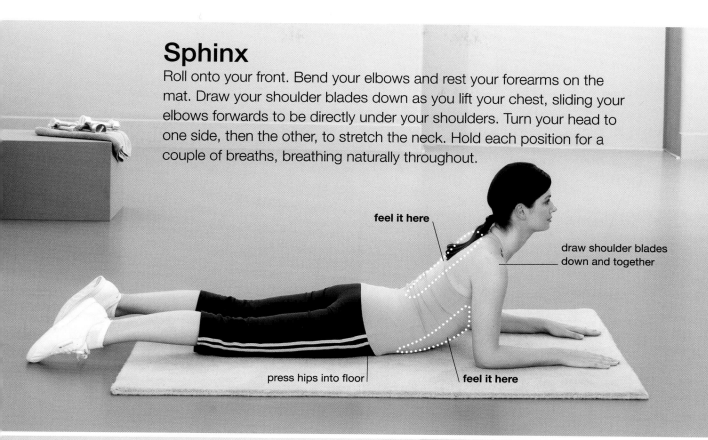

feel it here

draw shoulder blades down and together

press hips into floor

feel it here

Child's pose

Sit back on your heels and bend forwards, with your forehead to the floor and your arms stretching in front. Walk your hands to one side, keeping your head between your elbows, then stretch to the other side. With every exhale, let your body sink deeper.

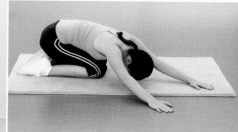

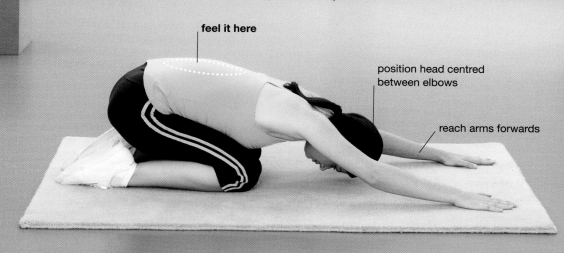

feel it here

position head centred between elbows

reach arms forwards

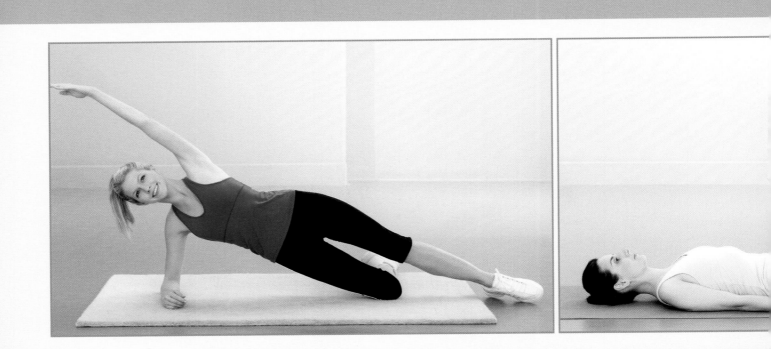

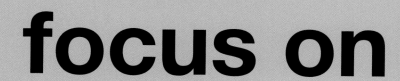

focus on

bum and thighs

Give your lower body a boost and pick 8–10 exercises to lift and shape your bum and firm up the thighs

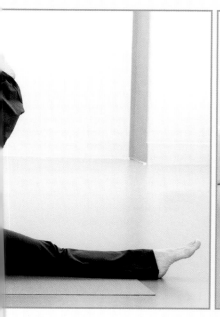

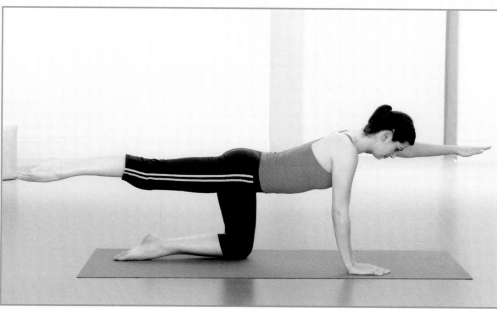

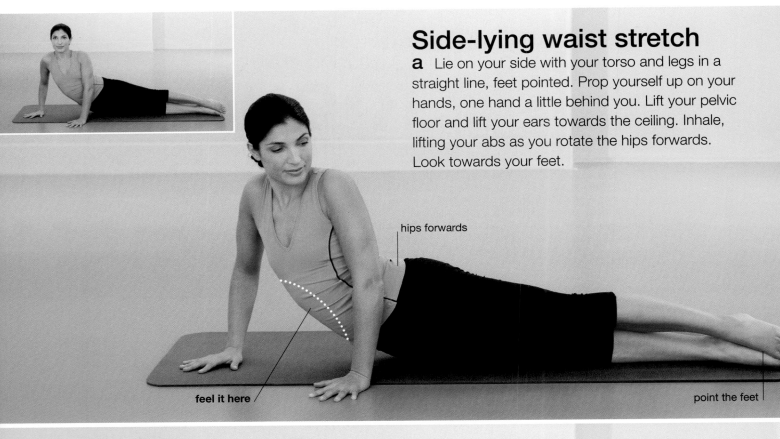

Side-lying waist stretch

a Lie on your side with your torso and legs in a straight line, feet pointed. Prop yourself up on your hands, one hand a little behind you. Lift your pelvic floor and lift your ears towards the ceiling. Inhale, lifting your abs as you rotate the hips forwards. Look towards your feet.

hips forwards

feel it here

point the feet

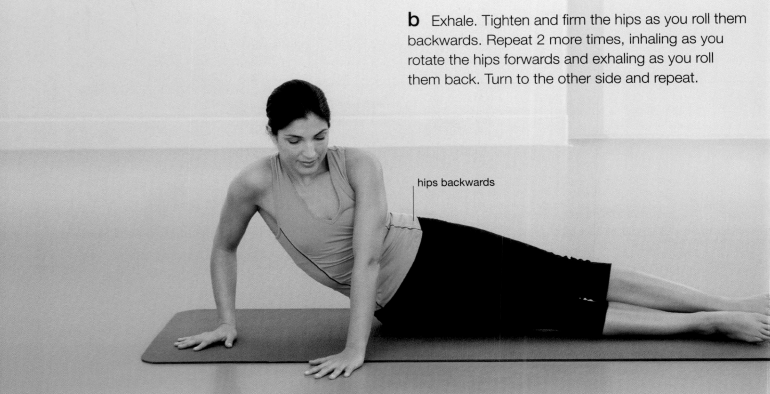

b Exhale. Tighten and firm the hips as you roll them backwards. Repeat 2 more times, inhaling as you rotate the hips forwards and exhaling as you roll them back. Turn to the other side and repeat.

hips backwards

Leg circles

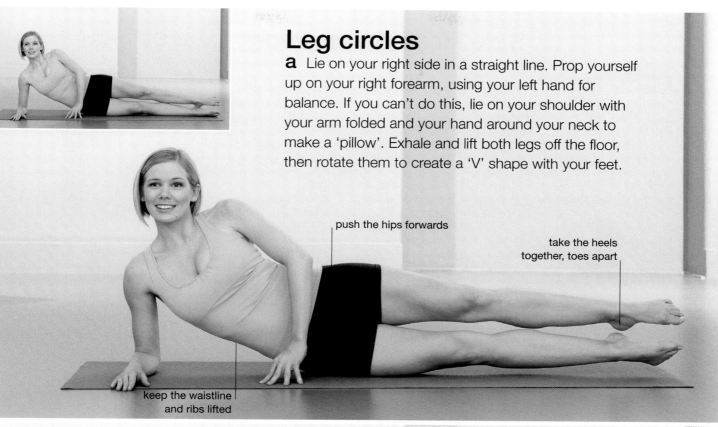

a Lie on your right side in a straight line. Prop yourself up on your right forearm, using your left hand for balance. If you can't do this, lie on your shoulder with your arm folded and your hand around your neck to make a 'pillow'. Exhale and lift both legs off the floor, then rotate them to create a 'V' shape with your feet.

push the hips forwards

take the heels together, toes apart

keep the waistline and ribs lifted

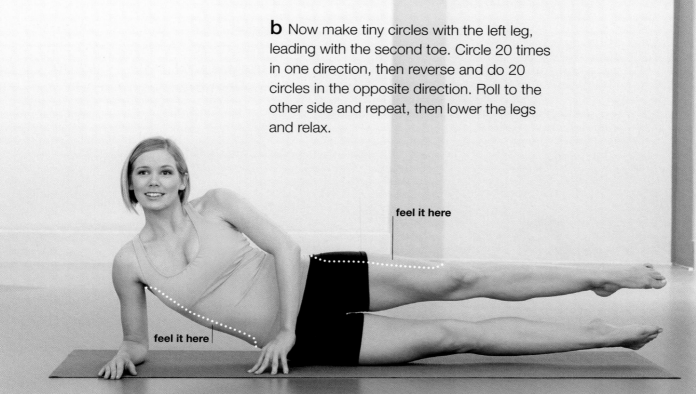

b Now make tiny circles with the left leg, leading with the second toe. Circle 20 times in one direction, then reverse and do 20 circles in the opposite direction. Roll to the other side and repeat, then lower the legs and relax.

feel it here

feel it here

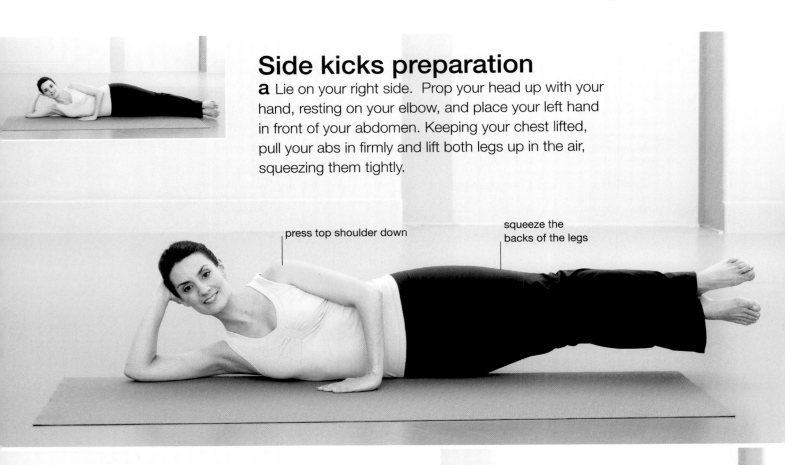

Side kicks preparation

a Lie on your right side. Prop your head up with your hand, resting on your elbow, and place your left hand in front of your abdomen. Keeping your chest lifted, pull your abs in firmly and lift both legs up in the air, squeezing them tightly.

press top shoulder down

squeeze the backs of the legs

b Without disrupting your posture, take your legs forwards and lower them with control. Your upper and lower body should make a 45° angle, with your hips and shoulders stacked one on top of the other.

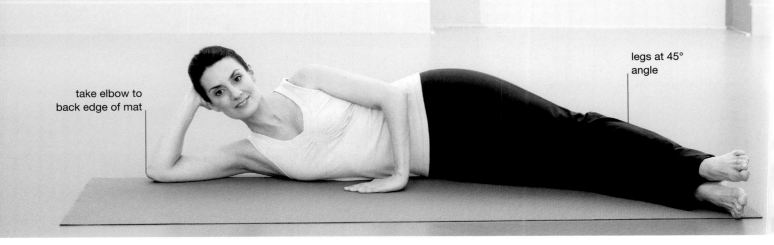

take elbow to back edge of mat

legs at 45° angle

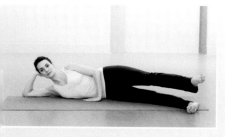

Side kicks front

a Keeping your upper and lower body at a 45° angle to each other, raise your left leg and slightly rotate it up to the ceiling. Keep your right foot solidly on the floor, slightly flexed and pressing down into the floor. Carry your leg forwards in a kicking motion, pulsing twice at the height of your kick.

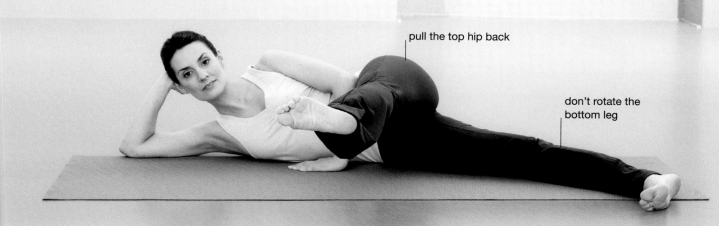

pull the top hip back

don't rotate the bottom leg

b Sweep the leg down and back behind the body, tightening the buttock muscles. Keep the upper body still and strong. Repeat a total of 6 times, then bring the leg back to its starting position.

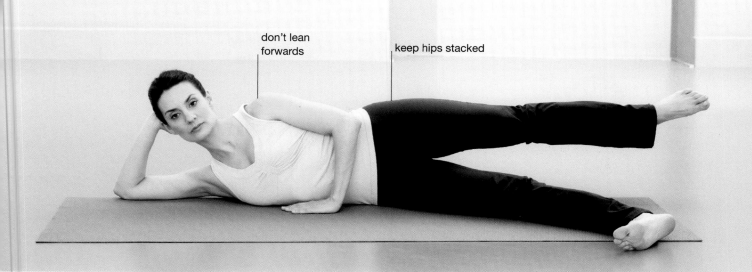

don't lean forwards

keep hips stacked

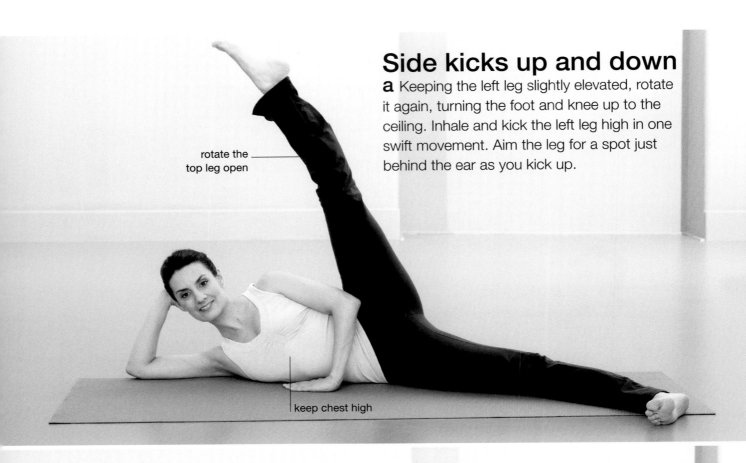

rotate the top leg open

keep chest high

Side kicks up and down

a Keeping the left leg slightly elevated, rotate it again, turning the foot and knee up to the ceiling. Inhale and kick the left leg high in one swift movement. Aim the leg for a spot just behind the ear as you kick up.

b Lower your leg, creating resistance as you go, for a count of 3. As your leg lowers, your abs should draw inwards and upwards. Lift your chest as you repeat 5 more times.

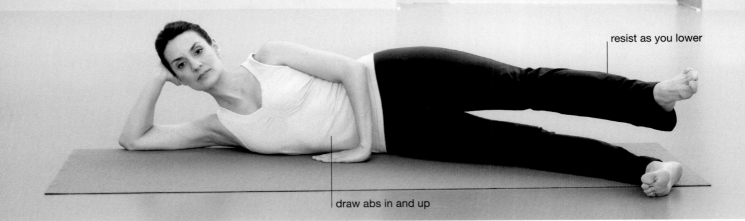

resist as you lower

draw abs in and up

Side kicks circles

a Remain lying on your side. Carry the top leg just in front of the bottom leg. It should feel very heavy at this point. Keep it rotated up to the sky with the ankle long.

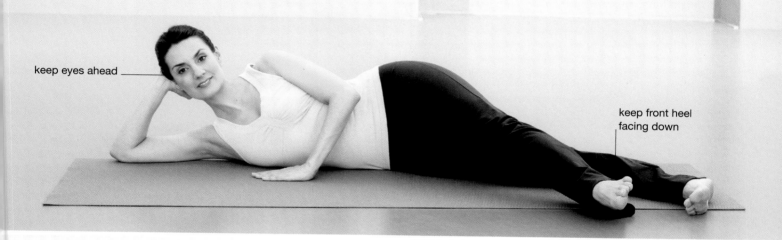

keep eyes ahead

keep front heel facing down

b Draw 10 tiny circles with the leg in the air without moving your body. Pause briefly. Switch immediately, taking the left leg back and reversing the circles. Keep the circles tiny and emphasize the downwards portion of the circle. Repeat 10 circles and pause before resting the left leg on the right.

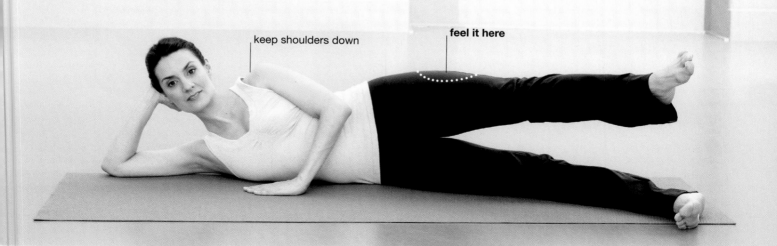

keep shoulders down

feel it here

Side kicks inner-thigh lifts

a Remain lying on your right side. Cross the left leg in front
of the right leg and take hold of the ankle. Place the left foot flat
on the floor with the knee and foot pointing down towards the
bottom foot. Now, flex the right foot and lift the entire right leg
just above the floor.

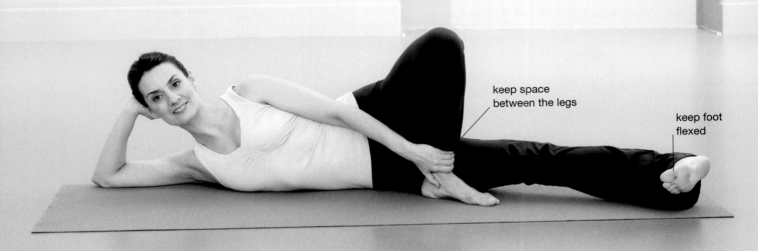

keep space
between the legs

keep foot
flexed

b Without hunching or collapsing, raise the right leg to its
highest point and lower it back to above the floor. Repeat 7
more times. On the last, remain at the highest point and perfect
the position by lengthening, straightening and rotating just a little
bit more. Finally, lower the leg with control.

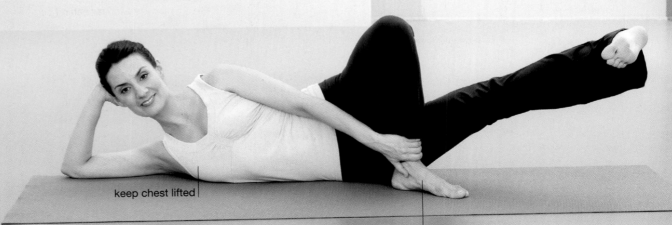

keep chest lifted

foot on mat angles down

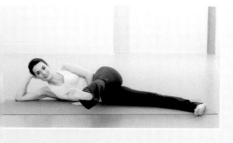

Side kicks bicycle

a Lie with the legs together at a 45° angle in front of you. Raise the left leg slightly. Swing it out in front of the body without hunching or rounding your back. Create a feeling of opposition by pulling back, or retracting, the left hip behind you slightly. Bend your left knee in towards your left shoulder.

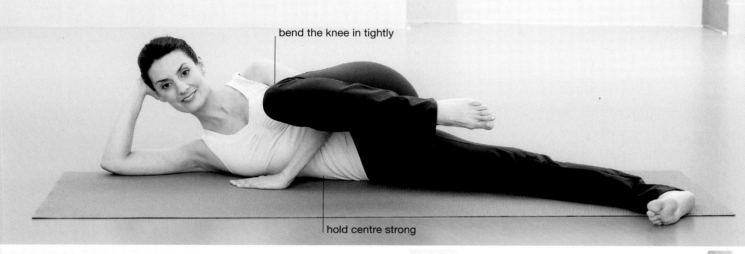

bend the knee in tightly

hold centre strong

b Sweep the left knee down to the right knee, then extend it behind you. Pull your waist up in opposition to the leg reaching back. Repeat 2 more times, then return the leg to its start position. Reverse direction, taking the leg backwards then forwards. Do this 3 times, then turn over to lie on your left side and repeat.

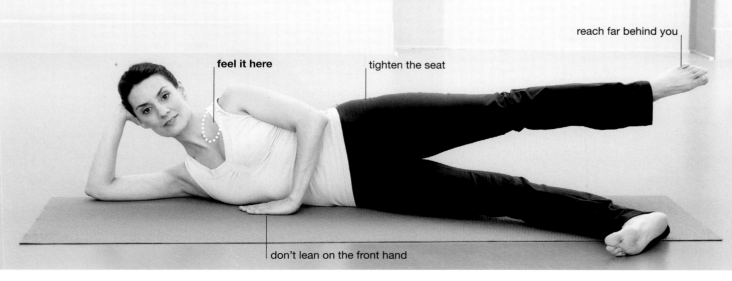

reach far behind you

feel it here

tighten the seat

don't lean on the front hand

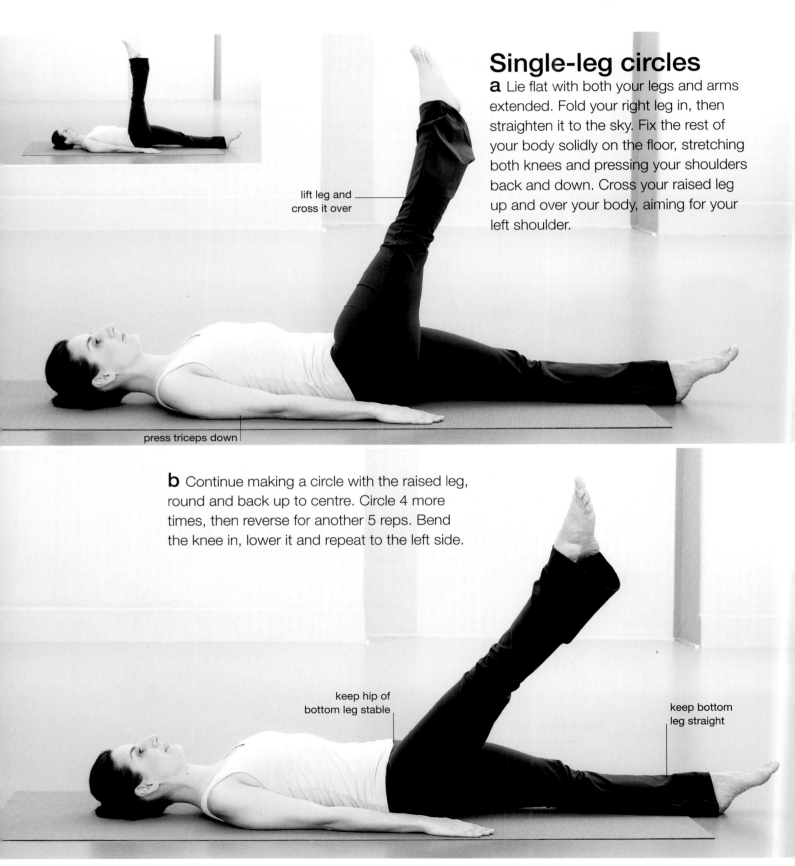

Single-leg circles

a Lie flat with both your legs and arms extended. Fold your right leg in, then straighten it to the sky. Fix the rest of your body solidly on the floor, stretching both knees and pressing your shoulders back and down. Cross your raised leg up and over your body, aiming for your left shoulder.

lift leg and cross it over

press triceps down

b Continue making a circle with the raised leg, round and back up to centre. Circle 4 more times, then reverse for another 5 reps. Bend the knee in, lower it and repeat to the left side.

keep hip of bottom leg stable

keep bottom leg straight

Single-leg stretch

a Lie flat with both knees bent into your chest. Before you curl up, be sure your shoulders are parallel to your hips and and activate your abs.

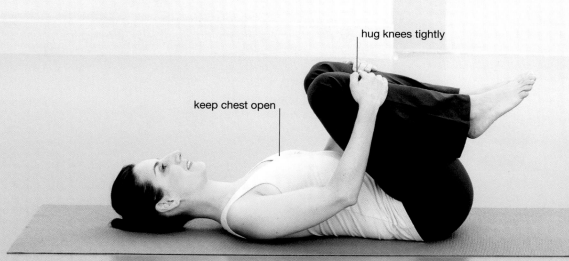

hug knees tightly

keep chest open

b Curl the upper body off the mat and hold the left leg, reaching the left hand to the ankle and the other to the knee. Extend the right leg 45°. Control the torso as you switch legs, inhaling on one side and exhaling on the other. Continue switching for 8 reps. Bend both knees to finish, then lie flat.

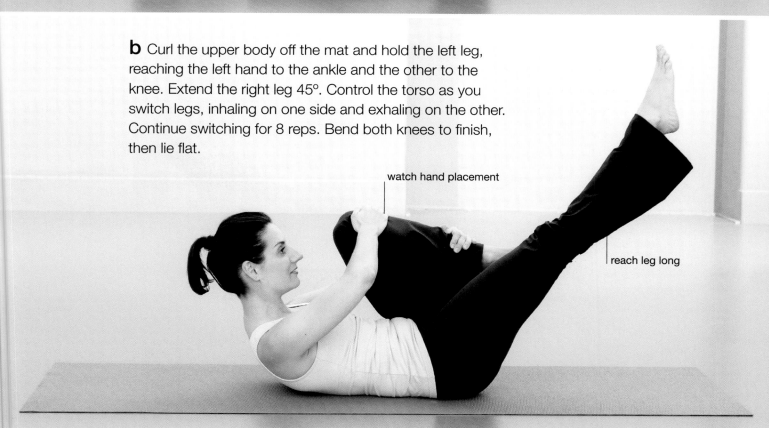

watch hand placement

reach leg long

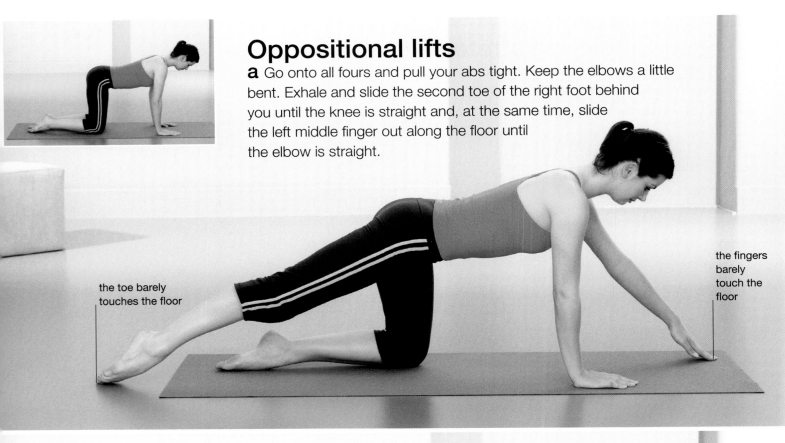

Oppositional lifts

a Go onto all fours and pull your abs tight. Keep the elbows a little bent. Exhale and slide the second toe of the right foot behind you until the knee is straight and, at the same time, slide the left middle finger out along the floor until the elbow is straight.

the toe barely touches the floor

the fingers barely touch the floor

b Exhale and take the right foot and left hand up until they are horizontal. Stay and inhale, then exhale as you lower just to touch the fingertip and tops of the toes to the floor. Reach out and away from the torso to repeat. Breathe and lower. Repeat on the other side.

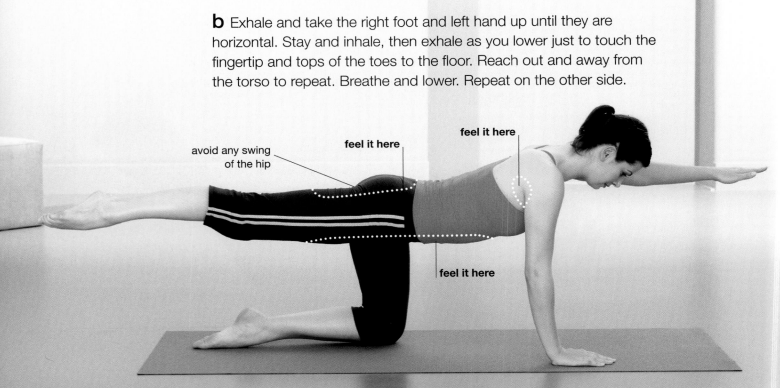

avoid any swing of the hip

feel it here

feel it here

feel it here

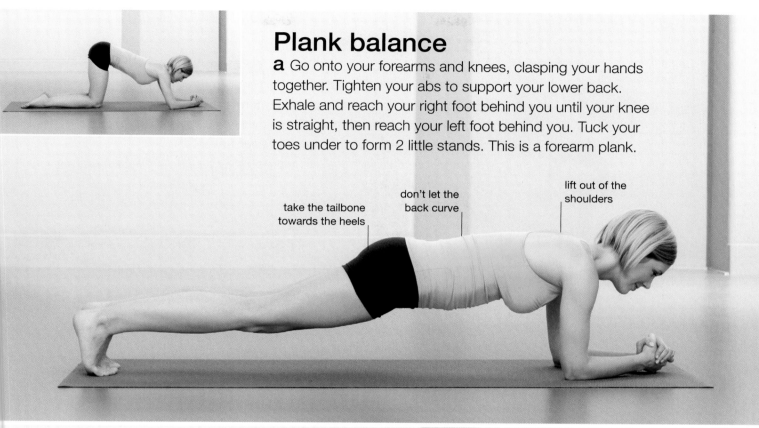

Plank balance

a Go onto your forearms and knees, clasping your hands together. Tighten your abs to support your lower back. Exhale and reach your right foot behind you until your knee is straight, then reach your left foot behind you. Tuck your toes under to form 2 little stands. This is a forearm plank.

lift out of the shoulders

don't let the back curve

take the tailbone towards the heels

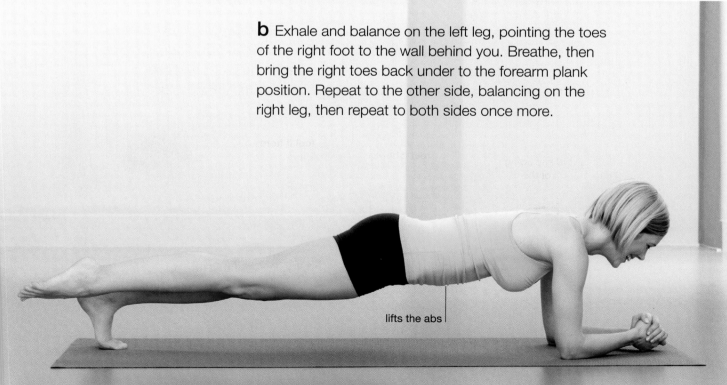

b Exhale and balance on the left leg, pointing the toes of the right foot to the wall behind you. Breathe, then bring the right toes back under to the forearm plank position. Repeat to the other side, balancing on the right leg, then repeat to both sides once more.

lifts the abs

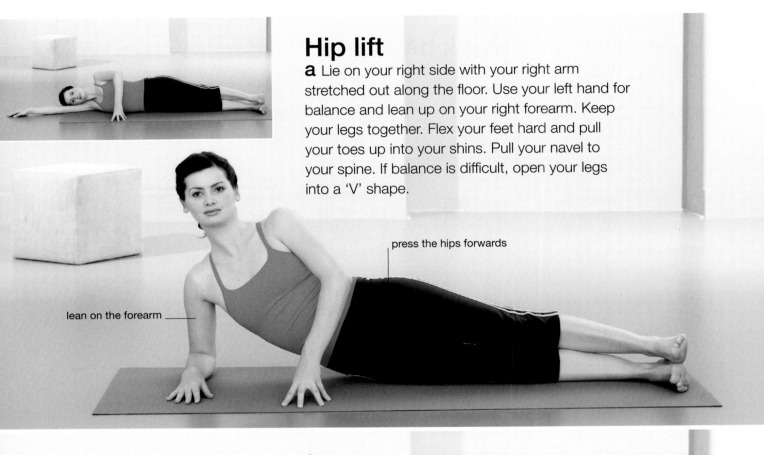

Hip lift

a Lie on your right side with your right arm stretched out along the floor. Use your left hand for balance and lean up on your right forearm. Keep your legs together. Flex your feet hard and pull your toes up into your shins. Pull your navel to your spine. If balance is difficult, open your legs into a 'V' shape.

press the hips forwards

lean on the forearm

b Inhale, then exhale and press downwards on the legs as you look down and lift the pelvis off the floor. Hold for a moment, then lower, but not completely. Repeat 3 more times, then repeat lying on the left side.

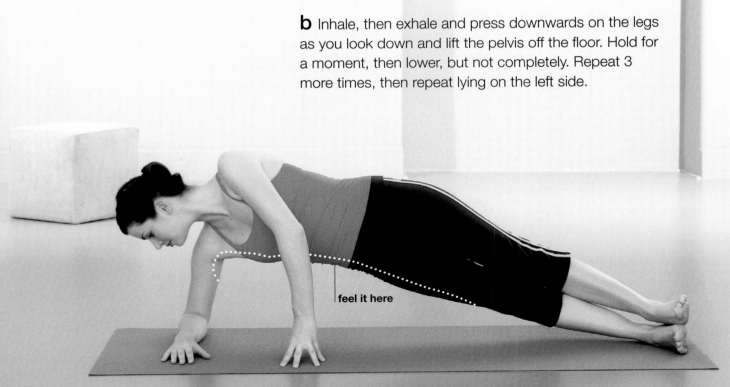

feel it here

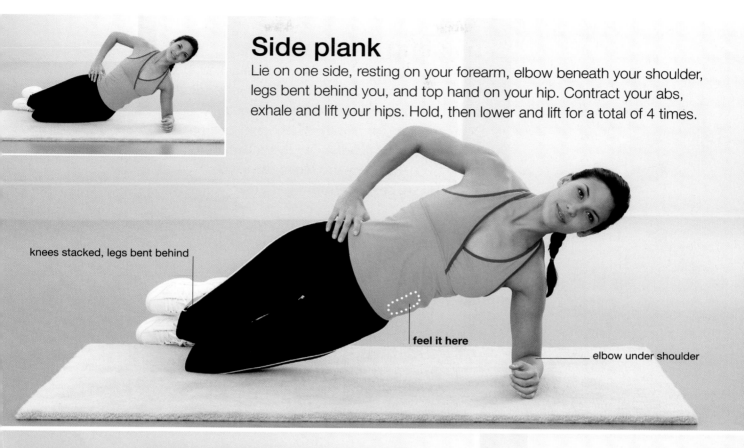

Side plank

Lie on one side, resting on your forearm, elbow beneath your shoulder, legs bent behind you, and top hand on your hip. Contract your abs, exhale and lift your hips. Hold, then lower and lift for a total of 4 times.

knees stacked, legs bent behind

feel it here

elbow under shoulder

Side plank with clam

Now add a challenging 'clam' by opening and closing your top knee 4 times. Keep your rib cage lifted and the lower shoulder down. Breathe naturally. Repeat Side plank and Side plank with clam lying on the other side.

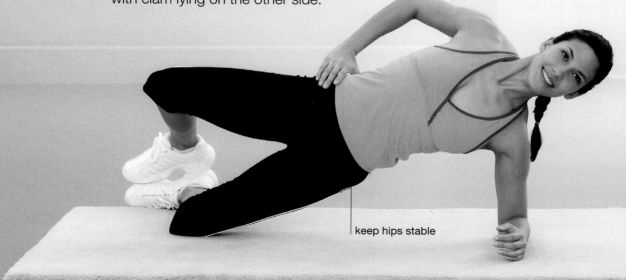

keep hips stable

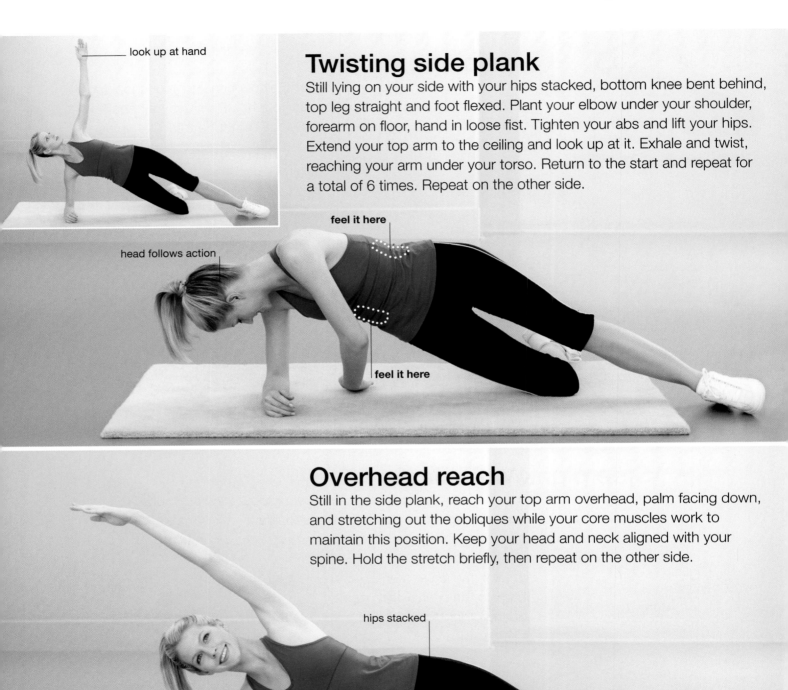

look up at hand

Twisting side plank

Still lying on your side with your hips stacked, bottom knee bent behind, top leg straight and foot flexed. Plant your elbow under your shoulder, forearm on floor, hand in loose fist. Tighten your abs and lift your hips. Extend your top arm to the ceiling and look up at it. Exhale and twist, reaching your arm under your torso. Return to the start and repeat for a total of 6 times. Repeat on the other side.

feel it here

head follows action

feel it here

Overhead reach

Still in the side plank, reach your top arm overhead, palm facing down, and stretching out the obliques while your core muscles work to maintain this position. Keep your head and neck aligned with your spine. Hold the stretch briefly, then repeat on the other side.

hips stacked

abs tight

rib cage lifted

Side stretch

Sit up and bend your knees to one side. Reach your opposite arm overhead, palm down. Stretch out all the muscles on the working side, then switch your legs around and repeat steps on the other side.

keep shoulder blade down

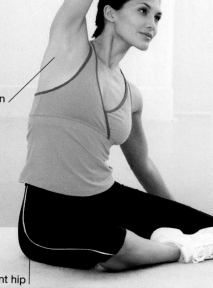

weight on front hip

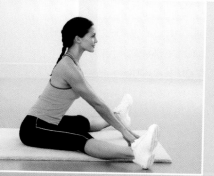

Wide 'V' stretch

Sit tall and open your legs in a wide 'V'. Lean forwards from your hips with your spine straight and reach your arms to centre. Keeping both your hips planted evenly on the floor, lift your spine, then turn your torso to face one leg and hold. Come back to the centre, then repeat on the other side.

spine straight

hips firmly planted

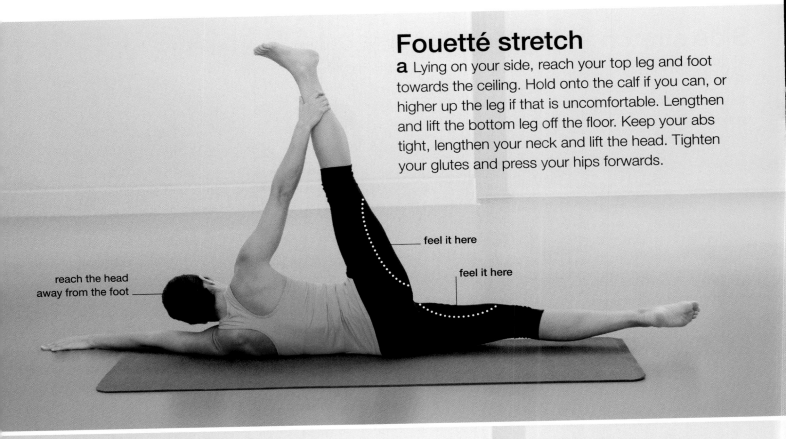

Fouetté stretch

a Lying on your side, reach your top leg and foot towards the ceiling. Hold onto the calf if you can, or higher up the leg if that is uncomfortable. Lengthen and lift the bottom leg off the floor. Keep your abs tight, lengthen your neck and lift the head. Tighten your glutes and press your hips forwards.

feel it here

feel it here

reach the head away from the foot

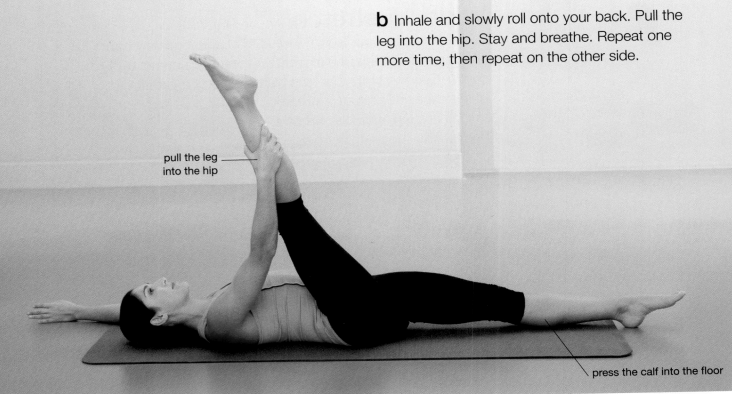

b Inhale and slowly roll onto your back. Pull the leg into the hip. Stay and breathe. Repeat one more time, then repeat on the other side.

pull the leg into the hip

press the calf into the floor

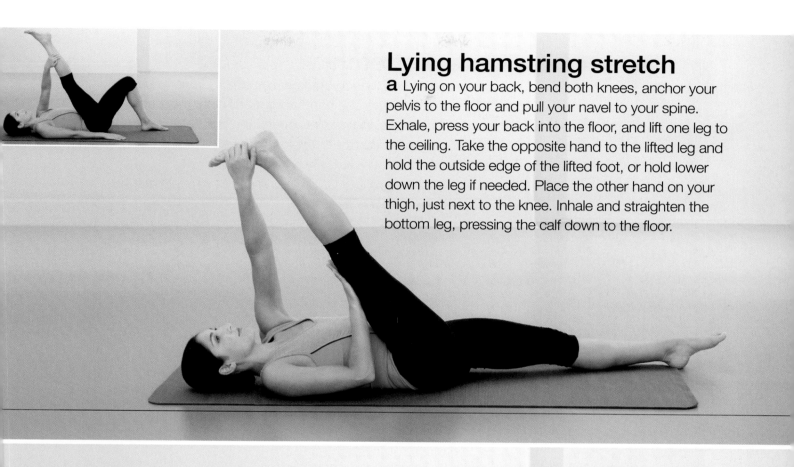

Lying hamstring stretch

a Lying on your back, bend both knees, anchor your pelvis to the floor and pull your navel to your spine. Exhale, press your back into the floor, and lift one leg to the ceiling. Take the opposite hand to the lifted leg and hold the outside edge of the lifted foot, or hold lower down the leg if needed. Place the other hand on your thigh, just next to the knee. Inhale and straighten the bottom leg, pressing the calf down to the floor.

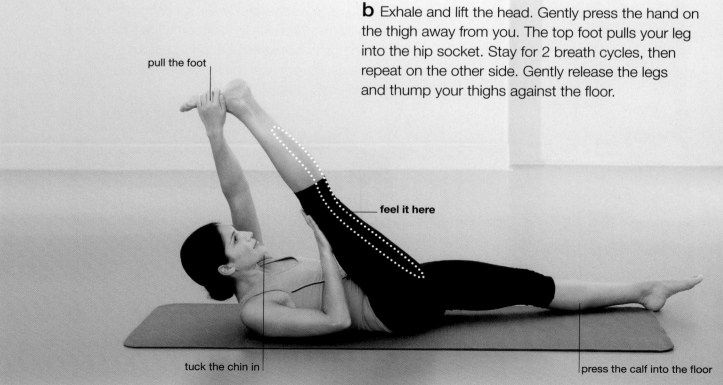

b Exhale and lift the head. Gently press the hand on the thigh away from you. The top foot pulls your leg into the hip socket. Stay for 2 breath cycles, then repeat on the other side. Gently release the legs and thump your thighs against the floor.

pull the foot

feel it here

tuck the chin in

press the calf into the floor

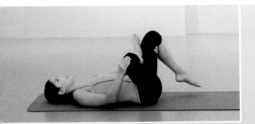

Figure 4 stretch

a Lying on your back, bend your knees and place one ankle on the other thigh. Place one hand underneath that thigh and the palm of the other hand on the knee of the crossed leg. Pull your abs tight to stabilize the spine. Inhale and pull the hand behind the thigh towards your chest.

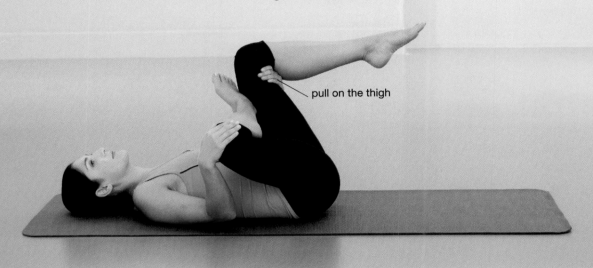

pull on the thigh

b Exhale and press the hand against the knee, away from your face, keeping the bent leg parallel to the floor. If the knee hurts, come out of the position, or loosen the posture. Repeat. Release both legs, thump your thighs, and breathe normally. Repeat on the other side.

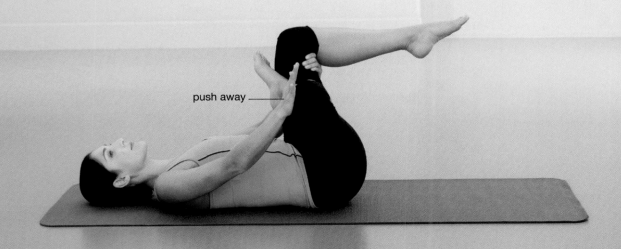

push away

Baby rocks

a Lie on your back. Exhale, press your back against the floor, and slowly slide your feet towards your hips. Lift your feet, one at a time, and hold onto them from outside your legs, keeping your knees bent. If you can't reach your feet, hold onto your shins.

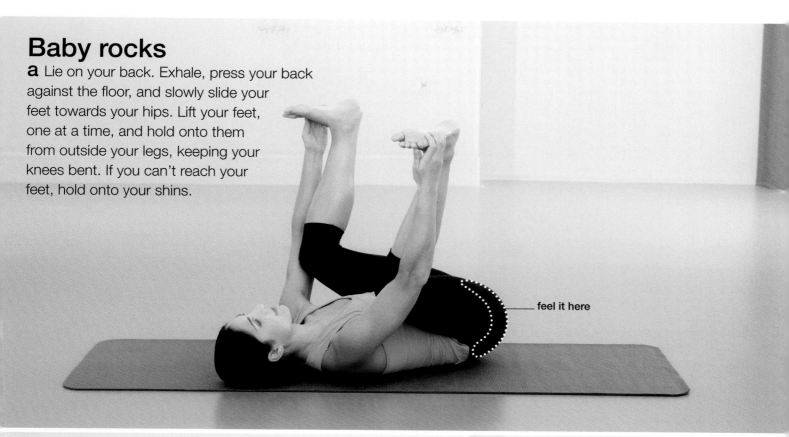

feel it here

b Inhale, pull one knee down towards the floor, and rock towards that side. Then, exhale and release to return to centre. Repeat, rocking to the other side, then repeat twice more.

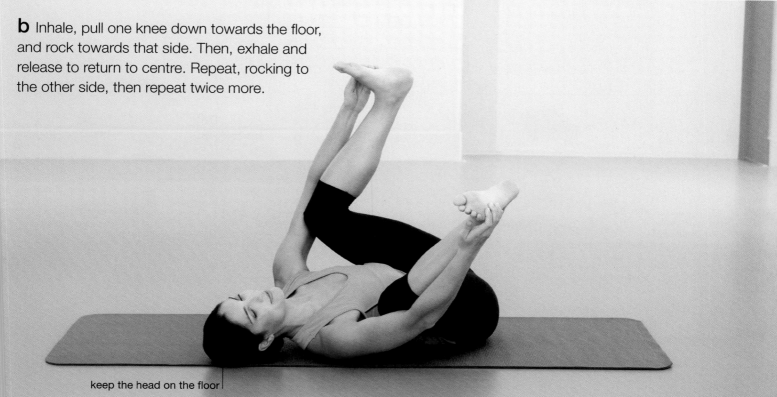

keep the head on the floor

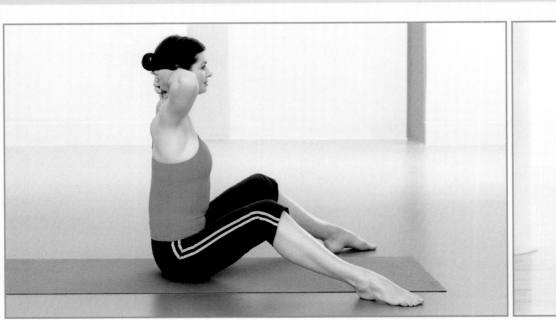
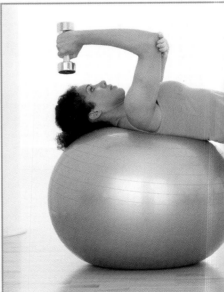

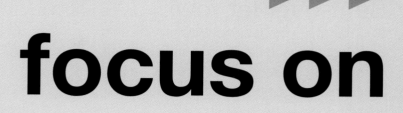

focus on

arms and back

Improve muscle tone and enhance your posture. Pick 8–10 exercises to bare arms with confidence and stand tall

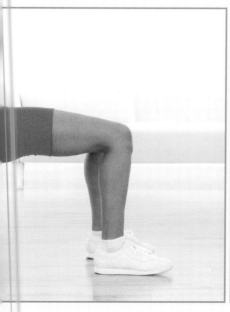

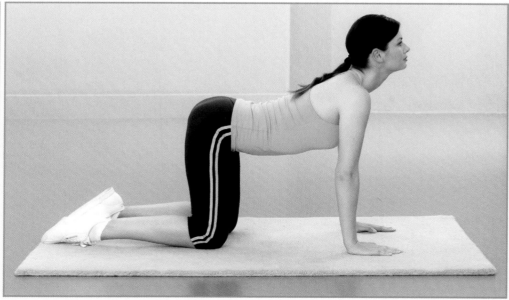

Bent-over lat row

a Stand with your feet hip width apart. Hold a free weight in each hand, arms at your sides, palms facing in. Bend forwards from the hips until your back is to the ceiling and your arms hang straight down under your shoulders. Keep your nose down.

b Draw your shoulder blades down and together. You can hold this position during the entire exercise or do it at the start of each rep. Inhale, then exhale and bend your arms to 90 degrees, pulling the weights up towards your waist. Pause, then inhale as you straighten your arms slowly to the start position. Do 1–2 sets of 10 reps, increasing the weight or number of reps as you progress.

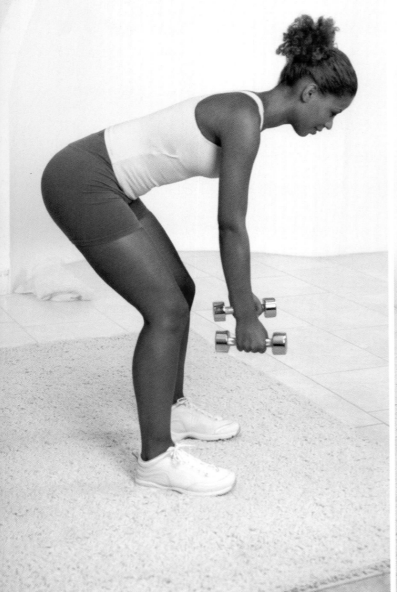

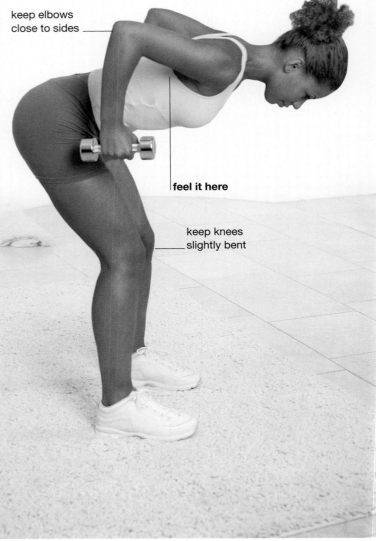

keep elbows close to sides

feel it here

keep knees slightly bent

Lat row

This exercise works the lats and the posterior deltoids, which are used for any pulling or lifting activity. Strengthening these muscles will make carrying your weekly shop much easier! Do 1–2 sets of 10 reps, increasing the band's resistance or number of reps as you progress.

Upper-back row

Along with the posterior deltoids, the upper-back row works the rhomboids and trapezius. Keep the band taut throughout your set. Do 1–2 sets of 10 reps, increasing the band's resistance or number of reps as you progress.

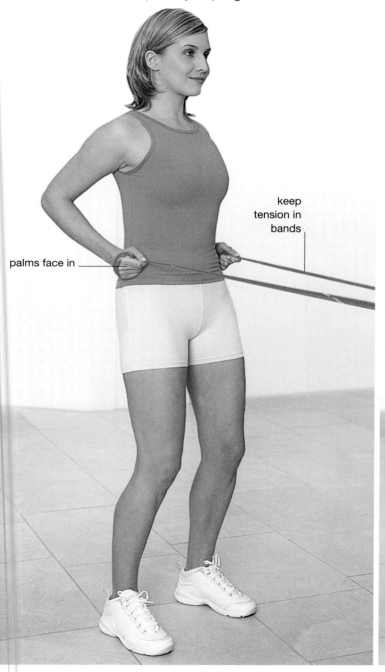

palms face in

keep tension in bands

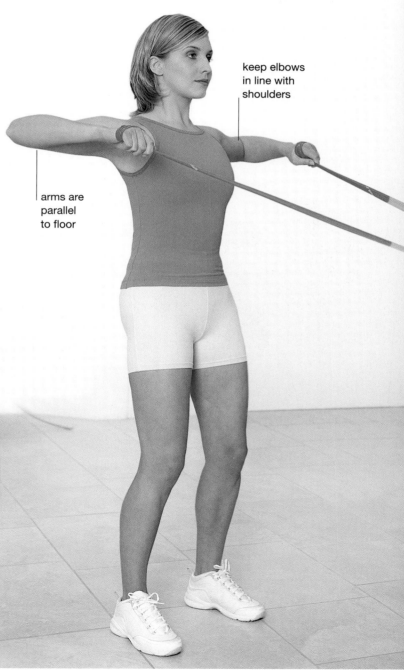

keep elbows in line with shoulders

arms are parallel to floor

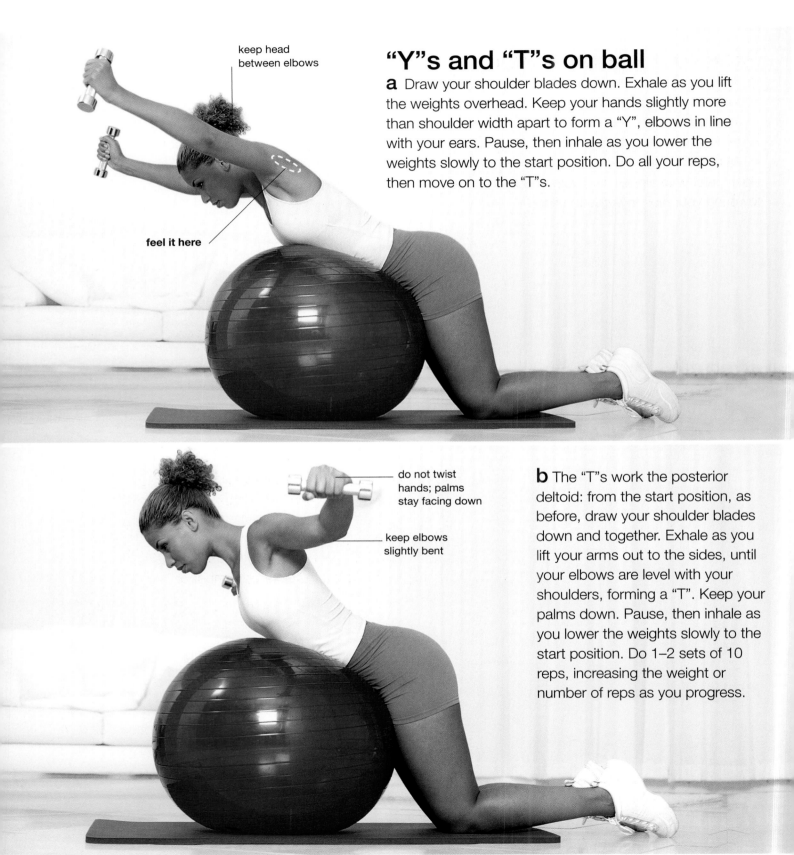

keep head
between elbows

feel it here

"Y"s and "T"s on ball

a Draw your shoulder blades down. Exhale as you lift the weights overhead. Keep your hands slightly more than shoulder width apart to form a "Y", elbows in line with your ears. Pause, then inhale as you lower the weights slowly to the start position. Do all your reps, then move on to the "T"s.

do not twist
hands; palms
stay facing down

keep elbows
slightly bent

b The "T"s work the posterior deltoid: from the start position, as before, draw your shoulder blades down and together. Exhale as you lift your arms out to the sides, until your elbows are level with your shoulders, forming a "T". Keep your palms down. Pause, then inhale as you lower the weights slowly to the start position. Do 1–2 sets of 10 reps, increasing the weight or number of reps as you progress.

Side-lying lateral raise

a To emphasize the medial deltoid, lie on your side on a mat or a well-padded surface. With hips stacked, shoulder to the ceiling, bend both knees 45 degrees forwards of the body. Rest your head on your bent arm, a small pillow, or a folded towel. Hold a free weight at your hip with your palm down, elbow straight. Draw your shoulder blade down. lowering your hips towards the floor.

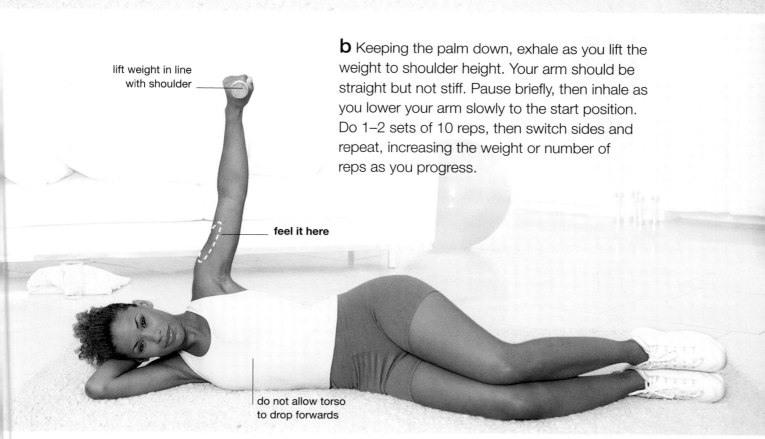

lift weight in line with shoulder

feel it here

do not allow torso to drop forwards

b Keeping the palm down, exhale as you lift the weight to shoulder height. Your arm should be straight but not stiff. Pause briefly, then inhale as you lower your arm slowly to the start position. Do 1–2 sets of 10 reps, then switch sides and repeat, increasing the weight or number of reps as you progress.

Front and side shoulder raise

a Stand with your feet parallel, hip width apart, knees soft. Hold a free weight in each hand, rms in front of your thighs, palms facing back. Pull your shoulder blades down and together.

b Breathe in, then as you exhale, lift both arms to the front, to shoulder height. Keep your wrists flat and your forearms parallel. Your arms should be straight but not stiff.

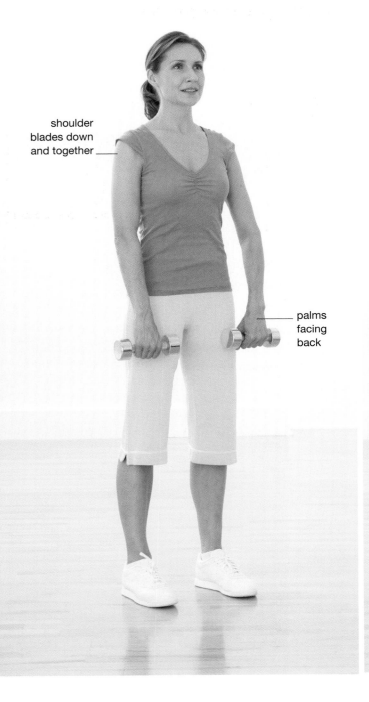

shoulder blades down and together

palms facing back

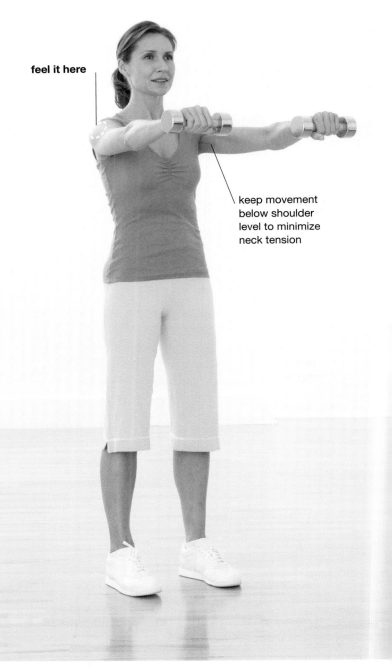

feel it here

keep movement below shoulder level to minimize neck tension

c Pause for a moment, then slowly lower your arms to the start position, keeping your shoulders back. Turn your arms, so that your palms now face in.

d Inhale, then, as you exhale, lift your arms out to the sides, to shoulder level (no higher), with your elbows in line with your shoulders. Keep your elbows slightly rounded, with palms facing down at the top of the movement. Inhale and slowly return to the start position. Do 1 set of 10 reps, increasing the weight or number of reps as you progress.

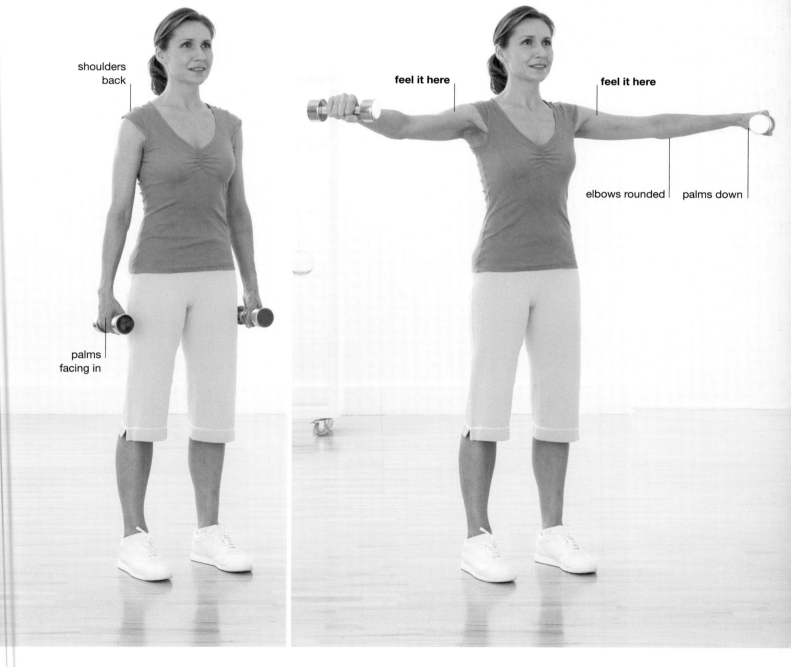

shoulders back

palms facing in

feel it here

feel it here

elbows rounded

palms down

Biceps "21"s

a Stand with your feet hip width apart. Hold a weight in each hand, palms facing forwards, arms straight. To work the lower range of motion, keep your elbows tight to your sides and exhale to lift the weights as high as your elbows. Do 7 reps. Inhale and slowly lower them.

b To work the upper range of motion, exhale to raise the weights from elbow height to shoulder height for 7 reps. Then do 7 reps working the full range of motion, raising the weights all the way up and down. Do 1 set, increasing the weight as you progress.

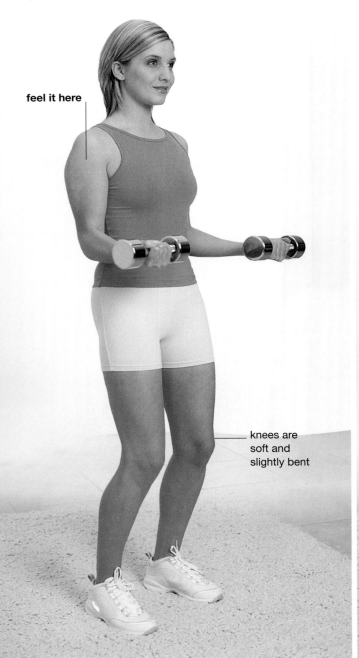

feel it here

knees are soft and slightly bent

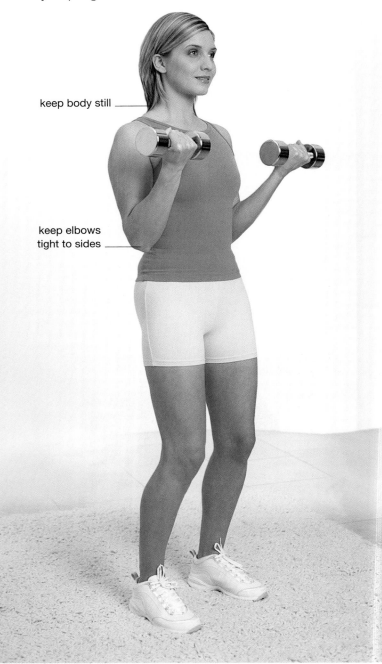

keep body still

keep elbows tight to sides

Double biceps curl

a Stand in a staggered lunge position with your right leg forward and right knee bent over the ankle. Anchor the band securely under the right foot, holding the ends of the band with your arms straight, palms facing forwards. Keep your wrists straight. Inhale.

b As you exhale, bend your elbows, pulling the band up and in towards your shoulders. Hold for a moment, then slowly release. If the band is a little short for your height, loop it under your thigh instead of anchoring it with your foot. Do 1–2 sets of 10 reps, increasing the band's resistance or number of reps as you progress.

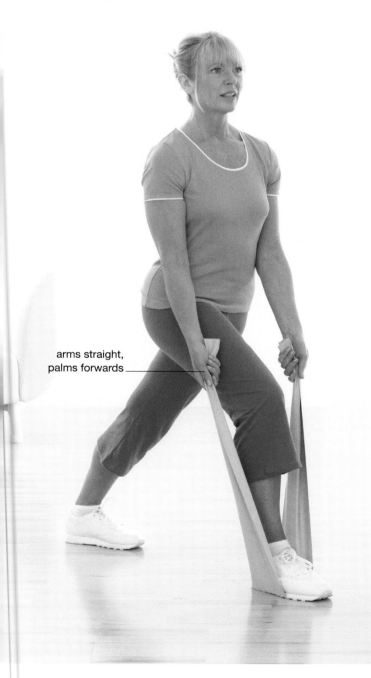

arms straight, palms forwards

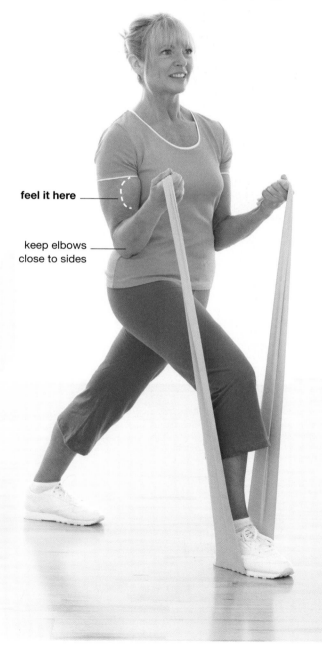

feel it here

keep elbows close to sides

Alternating biceps curl

a Stand with your feet parallel, hip width apart, knees soft. Hold a free weight in each hand, with your arms straight at your sides, wrists aligned with the forearms, palms facing in.

b Exhale and squeeze your upper arm as you bend your right elbow, lifting the weight towards your shoulder. To return, inhale and straighten your forearm fully, maintaining tension in the muscle. Do 1–2 sets of 10 reps, increasing the weight or number of reps as you progress.

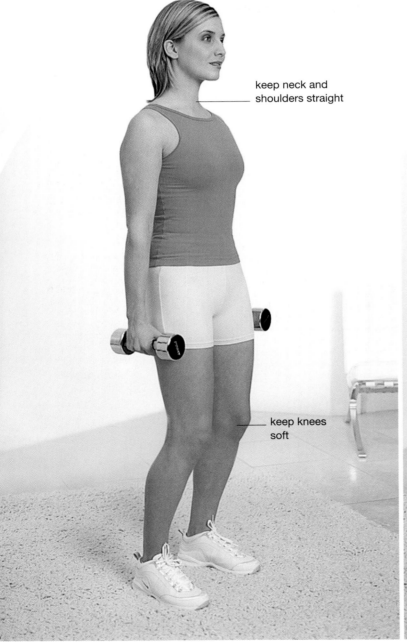

keep neck and shoulders straight

keep knees soft

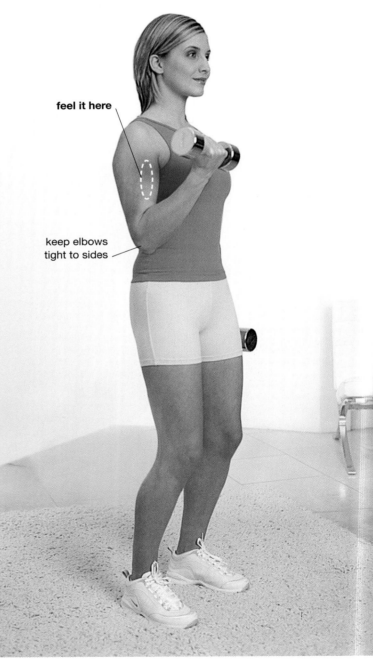

feel it here

keep elbows tight to sides

Concentration curl

a Holding a free weight in your left hand, sit forwards on a chair. Place your right hand on top of your right thigh and lean forwards from the hip. Brace the back of your left elbow against your left inner thigh and extend your left arm towards the floor, palm facing in. Inhale.

b As you exhale, bend your left elbow and contract the biceps to bring the weight up towards your shoulder. Pause, then slowly lower the weight to the start position, maintaining tension in the muscle. Do 1–2 sets of 10 reps, then switch sides and repeat. Increase the weight or number of reps as you progress.

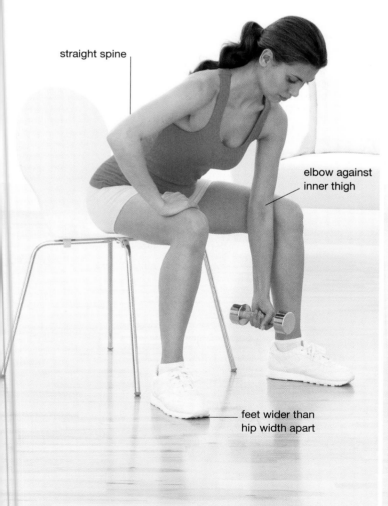

straight spine

elbow against inner thigh

feet wider than hip width apart

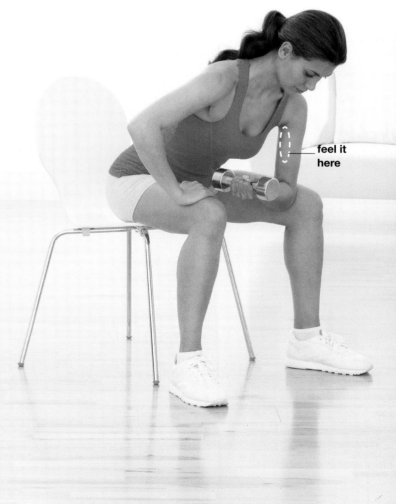

feel it here

Triceps kickback

a Stand with your feet parallel, hip width apart, knees bent. Bend forwards from the hip, keeping your spine straight. Holding weights in both hands with palms facing in, bend your elbows to 90 degrees and raise the upper arms so that they are parallel to the floor.

b Keeping your ab muscles tight, exhale as you extend your forearms behind you so that your arms are straight but not stiff. Pause and squeeze the backs of the upper arms. Inhale as you slowly return to the start position. Your head should remain in line with your spine throughout the exercise. Do 1–2 sets of 10 reps, increasing the weight or number of reps as you progress.

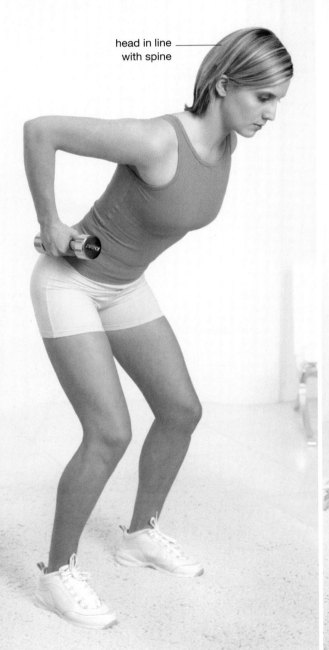

head in line with spine

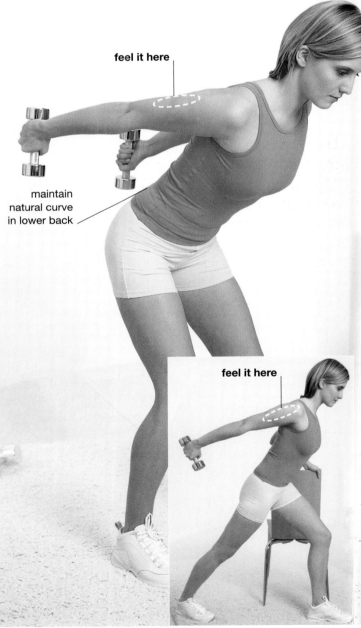

feel it here

maintain natural curve in lower back

feel it here

Triceps extension

a From a seated position on the ball, roll down into a bridge position with head, neck, and shoulders supported. Holding a free weight in your left hand, bend your elbow to 90 degrees. Brace the elbow with your right hand.

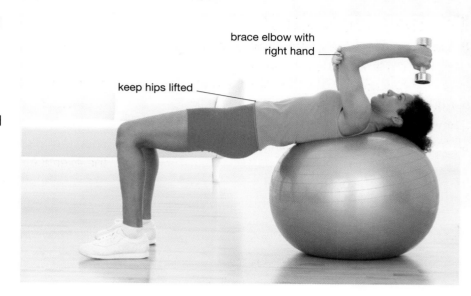

brace elbow with right hand

keep hips lifted

b Continuing to brace the back of your elbow with your right hand, exhale and straighten the arm to the ceiling. Do 1–2 sets of 10 reps, then switch sides and repeat. Increase the weight or number of reps as you progress.

palm in, wrist straight

head, neck, and shoulders supported

feel it here

Kneeling triceps kickback

a Kneeling on all fours, extend your left leg to the back at hip height. Holding a free weight in the right hand, bend your elbow to 90 degrees, anchoring your upper arm close to your side, parallel to the floor.

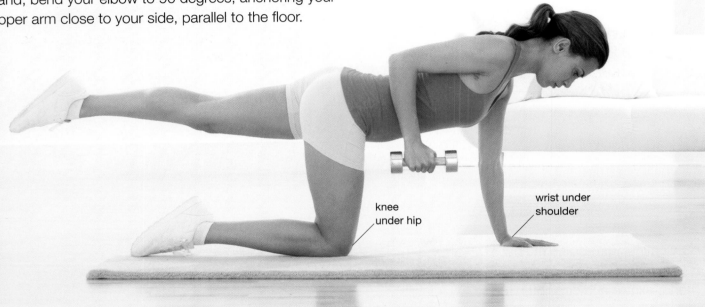

knee under hip

wrist under shoulder

b Exhale and straighten your right arm to the back, without locking the elbow, then return to the start position with the elbow bent at 90 degrees. Do 1–2 sets of 10 reps, then switch sides and repeat. Increase the weight or number of reps as you progress.

palm in, wrist straight

feel it here

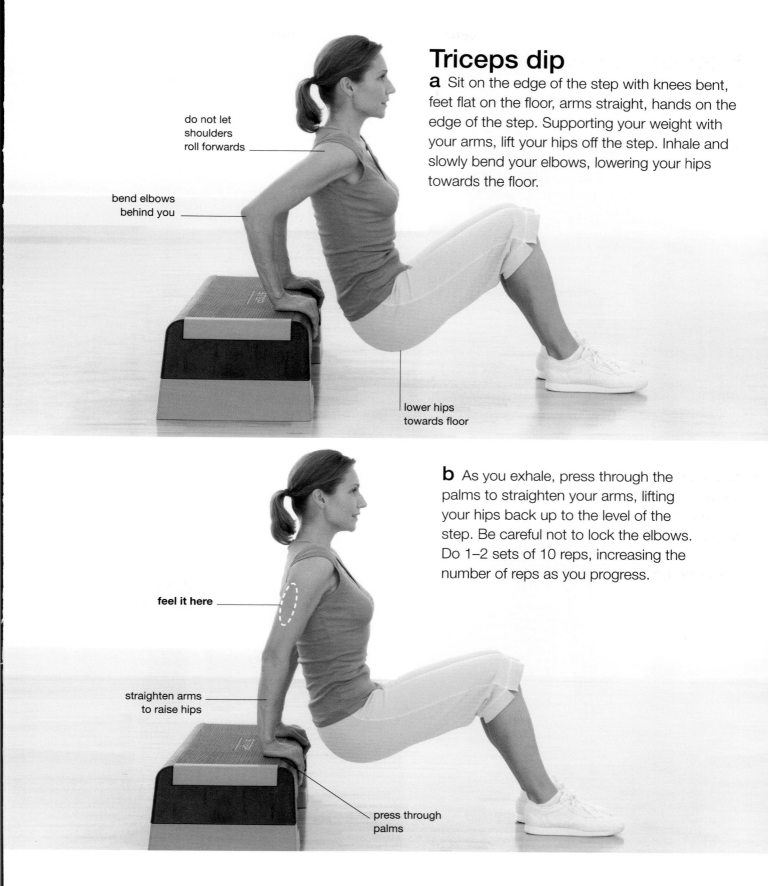

do not let
shoulders
roll forwards

bend elbows
behind you

lower hips
towards floor

Triceps dip

a Sit on the edge of the step with knees bent, feet flat on the floor, arms straight, hands on the edge of the step. Supporting your weight with your arms, lift your hips off the step. Inhale and slowly bend your elbows, lowering your hips towards the floor.

feel it here

straighten arms
to raise hips

press through
palms

b As you exhale, press through the palms to straighten your arms, lifting your hips back up to the level of the step. Be careful not to lock the elbows. Do 1–2 sets of 10 reps, increasing the number of reps as you progress.

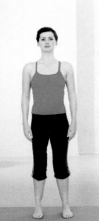

Shoulder circles

a With your legs shoulder-width apart, reach both arms overhead and clasp your fingers. Lengthen your tailbone towards the ground. Circle your arms, imagining making 4 circles on the ceiling with your hands. Return to centre.

b Again, lift up and out of the waist and tighten the waist. Lengthen the tailbone. Reverse the movement with the hands, imagining making 4 more circles on the ceiling. Bring the arms down.

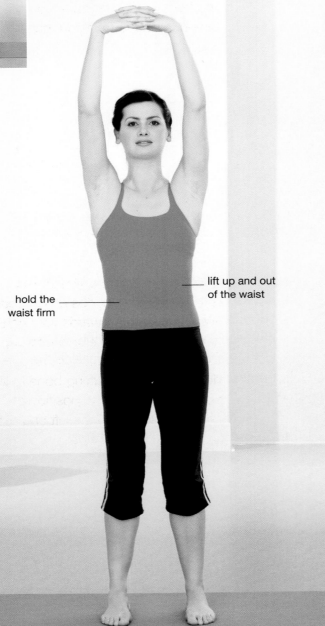

hold the waist firm

lift up and out of the waist

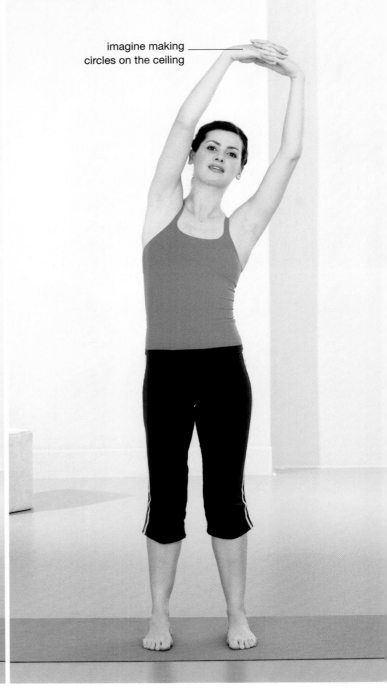

imagine making circles on the ceiling

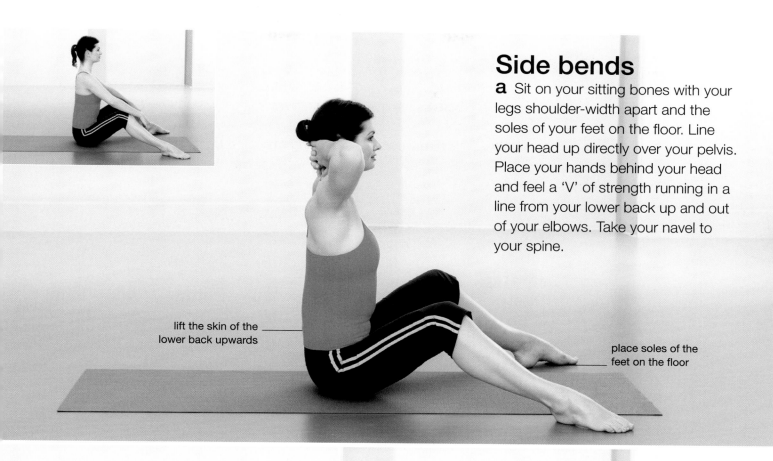

Side bends

a Sit on your sitting bones with your legs shoulder-width apart and the soles of your feet on the floor. Line your head up directly over your pelvis. Place your hands behind your head and feel a 'V' of strength running in a line from your lower back up and out of your elbows. Take your navel to your spine.

lift the skin of the lower back upwards

place soles of the feet on the floor

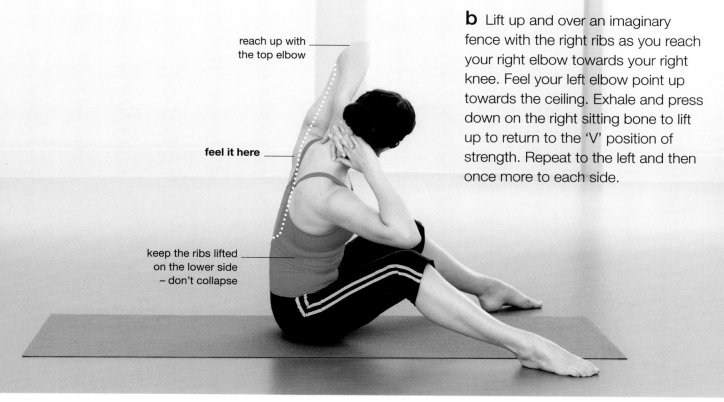

b Lift up and over an imaginary fence with the right ribs as you reach your right elbow towards your right knee. Feel your left elbow point up towards the ceiling. Exhale and press down on the right sitting bone to lift up to return to the 'V' position of strength. Repeat to the left and then once more to each side.

reach up with the top elbow

feel it here

keep the ribs lifted on the lower side – don't collapse

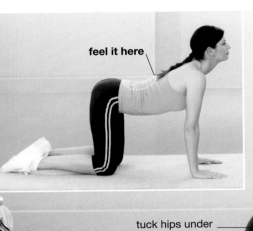

feel it here

Spinal arch

Come to all fours, knees under hips. Lift your head and hips up (inset). Then arch your spine, rounding it up to the ceiling by tucking your hips under and dropping your head between your arms. Alternate this with spinal curve (inset), repeating for a total of 3 times.

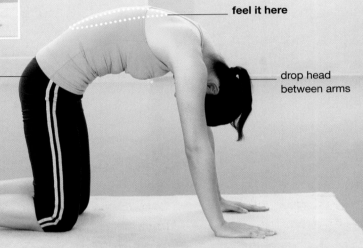

feel it here

tuck hips under

drop head between arms

Child's pose

Sit back, reaching your hips towards your heels, at the same time rounding forward and extending your arms in front of you until your head rests on the floor. Keep your elbows off the floor to get the best stretch. Sink down into the position, holding for 3 deep breath cycles and sinking deeper into the position with each exhalation.

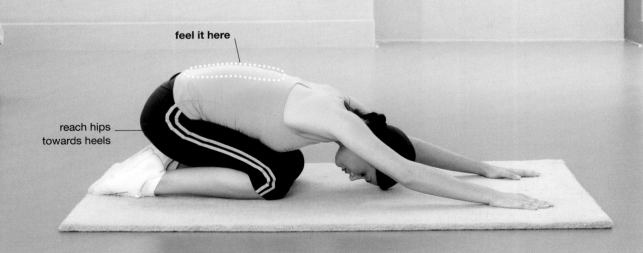

feel it here

reach hips towards heels

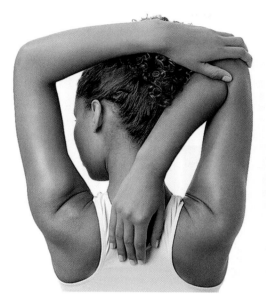

Triceps stretch

Raise one elbow to the ceiling and reach down your spine. Use the other arm to pull back gently on the elbow. Hold for 10 seconds on each side.

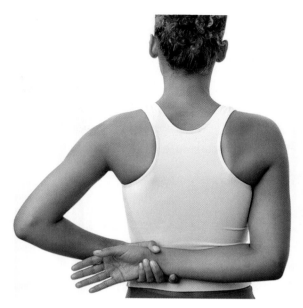

Anterior-deltoid stretch

Put one arm behind you and take it by the wrist. Gently pull the back arm across the back. Hold for 10 seconds on each side.

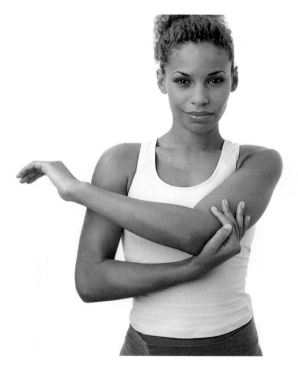

Posterior-deltoid stretch

Draw your shoulder blades down and together. Gently pull one arm across your chest with the other hand above the elbow. Hold for 10 seconds on each side.

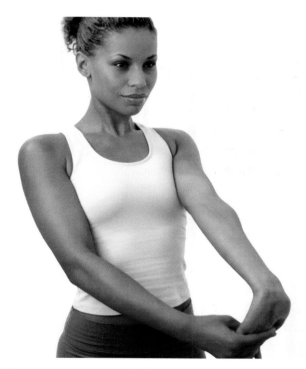

Biceps and forearm stretch

Extend one arm in front of you with the palm up. With the other hand, pull back on the palm. Hold for 10 seconds on each side.

144 acknowledgments ▶▶▶

Publisher's acknowledgments

Dorling Kindersley would like to thank photographer Ruth Jenkinson and her assistants, Ann Burke, James McNaught, Carly Churchill, and Vic Churchill; sweatyBetty for the loan of some of the exercise clothing; Viv Reily at Touch Studios; models Jacqui Freeman, Carla Collins, Kerry Jay, Rhona Crewe, Sam Magee, Tara Lee, and Samantha Johannesson; Rachel Jones, Brigitta Smart, Roisin Donaghy, and Victoria Barnes for hair and make up; YogaMatters for the loan of the mat and other equipment; Anna Toombs and David Robinson of TR Balance for additional training support. Project editors Helen Murray and Hilary Mandleberg; Senior editors Jennifer Latham, Jo Godfrey Wood; Project art editors Anne Fisher, Ruth Hope, and Helen McTeer; Senior art editors Peggy Sadler, Miranda Harvey, and Susan Downing.

about the authors ▶▶▶

Joan Pagano

Joan Pagano is a fitness expert and the owner of Joan Pagano Fitness in New York City. Former trainer to Jacqueline Onassis and Caroline Kennedy, Joan has specialized in strength training for women since 1988. Through her work she has created hundreds of training programmes custom-designed for individuals, groups, fitness facilities, schools, hospitals, and corporations. Joan is an authority on the benefits of exercise for women's health and focuses on issues such as pregnancy, menopause, osteoporosis, and breast cancer, as well as strength training through the decades. Certified as a Health and Fitness Specialist by the American College of Sports Medicine (ACSM), Joan is also a spokesperson for IDEA Health & Fitness Association, the world's largest association for fitness and wellness professionals. She is a Phi beta Kappa, cum laude graduate of Connecticut College and a member of Shaker Heights High School's Hall of Fame. Joan is the proud finisher of seven marathons.

Suzanne Martin

Suzanne Martin is a doctor of physical therapy and a gold-certified Pilates expert. A former dancer, she is a Master trainer certified by the American Council on Exercise. She is also well known as an educational presenter within the world of Pilates, dance, and physical therapy. Suzanne is the lead physical therapist for the Smuin Ballet in San Francisco and maintains a private practice, Total Body Development, in California.

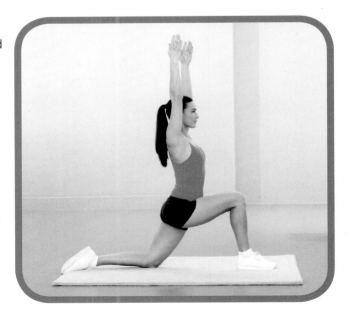

Alycea Ungaro

Alycea Ungaro, PT, is the owner of Alycea Ungaro's Real Pilates in New York City and the author several best-selling Pilates titles. Alycea's personal mission is to make Pilates available to everyone regardless of age, fitness level, or location.